FOUNDATIONS OF MANUAL LYMPH DRAINAGE

FOUNDATIONS OF MANUAL LYMPH DRAINAGE

Michael Földi, MD, and

Roman Strößenreuther, MD

THIRD EDITION

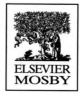

ELSEVIER
MOSBY

ELSEVIER
MOSBY

11830 Westline Industrial Drive
St. Louis, Missouri 63146

NOTICE

Massage therapy is an ever-changing field. Standard safety precautions
must be followed, but as new research and clinical experience broaden
our knowledge, changes in treatment and drug therapy may become
necessary or appropriate. Readers are advised to check the most current
product information provided by the manufacturer of each drug to be
administered to verify the recommended dose, the method and duration
of administration, and contraindications. It is the responsibility of the
licensed prescriber, relying on experience and knowledge of the patient,
to determine dosages and the best treatment for each individual patient.
Neither the publisher nor the author assumes any liability for any injury
and/or damage to persons or property arising from this publication.
The Publisher

International Standard Book Number 0-323-03064-5

Acquisitions Editor: Kellie White
Developmental Editor: Kim Fons
Publishing Services Manager: Patricia Tannian
Design Manager: Gail Morey Hudson

Printed in the United States of America

Last digit is the print number: 9   8   7   6   5   4   3   2   1

About the Authors

Michael Földi, MD, studied medicine in Hungary and went on to become Director of the II. University Medical Clinic in Szeged, Hungary. Today he is APL Professor at the University of Freiburg, Germany. As a student he developed an intense interest in lymphology, which was to become his specialty in later years. In 1986 at Hinterzarten in the Black Forest of Germany, he founded the Földi Clinic, a specialist clinic for lymphology, where he is active today as an advisor. His outstanding work and numerous publications have made him a founder and pioneer in lymphology. The numerous honorary memberships and awards he has received from national and international lymphology associations attest to the high regard in which he is held in this field.

Roman Strößenreuther, MD, completed his training as masseur/balneotherapist between 1981 and 1983. He worked as lymph drainage therapist, as assistant instructor, and later as technical instructor at the Földi Clinic for Lymphology and at the Földi Clinic's teaching institute, the Földi School. Subsequently he was active in various clinics and practices. From 1990 to 1996 he studied medicine in Munich and then worked as a physician in Gera and Freising, Germany. Since 1999 he has been the head of the Lymphangiology Department at the Freising-Moosburg hospital.

Preface

This text, now in a third, expanded edition, was designed to instruct physiotherapy and massage students in forms of massage therapy that include manual lymph drainage (MLD). Our intention in this work is to convey the scientific foundations and the principles of the MLD technique; we assume that the reader already has a knowledge of anatomy, histology, and the cardiovascular system.

Michael Földi, MD
Roman H.K. Strößenreuther, MD

ABBREVIATIONS

CBP	Capillary blood pressure
COP$_i$	Colloidal osmotic pressure in interstitial fluid
COP$_p$	Colloidal osmotic pressure in blood plasma
ERP	Effective reabsorption pressure
EUP	Effective ultrafiltration pressure
IP	Interstitial pressure

ILLUSTRATION CREDITS

A number in square brackets at the end of a figure legend indicates the source of the figure.

Source Number	Source
1	Földi M, Kubik S: *Lehrbuch der lymphologie,* ed 3, Stuttgart, 1993, Gustav Fischer Verlag.
2	Földi M, Földi E: *Das lymphödem,* ed 6, Stuttgart, 1993, Gustav Fischer Verlag.
3	Susanne Adler, Lubeck, Germany
4	Gerda Raichle, Ulm, Germany
5	Roman Strößenreuther, MD, Munich, Germany
6	Stefan Kubik, MD, Zurich, Switzerland
7	Michael Földi, MD, Hinterzarten, Germany
8	P.C. Scriba, MD, Munich, Germany

Contents

1 Anatomy of the Lymph Vessel System

Important tasks of the lymph vessel system are the drainage and transport of interstitial fluid or lymph.

The lymph vessel system is a component of the lymphatic system, which also includes the lymphatic organs (thymus, spleen, tonsils, etc.). The most important task of the lymph vessels is the drainage and transport of interstitial fluid, along with various substances contained in it, into the venous blood circulation.

The lymph vessels of the small intestine are capable of absorbing and transporting food fats away from the intestine. Furthermore, the lymphatic system is an important component of the immune defense system.

The goal of **manual lymph drainage** and **complete decongestive therapy** is to improve or restore lymph drainage that has become impaired. To apply these therapeutic methods successfully, the therapist must master the anatomy, physiology, and pathophysiology of the lymphatic system.

1.1 LYMPH VESSEL SYSTEM

The lymph vessel system is a drainage system. It transports lymph into the venous blood circulation. As in the veins, flap valves in the large lymph vessels ensure directionality of flow.

❶ Although the lymph vessels run broadly parallel to the blood vessels and have a similar wall construction, the blood and lymph vessels are different in several important ways (Fig. 1.1):

Unlike the blood vessels, the lymph vessels:
- Are not a component of a closed circuit
- Do not have a central pump comparable to the heart
- Have interposed lymph nodes

- **No closed circuit:** Contrary to the blood circulation, the lymph vessels form only half a circuit. They begin in the periphery with the so-called initial lymph vessels (lymph capillaries) and end by exiting into the large blood vessels of the venous blood circulation, near the heart.
- **No "central pump":** In the blood vessel system, the heart functions as a driver for the circulation of blood through the large and small blood vessels. The heart carries the

1

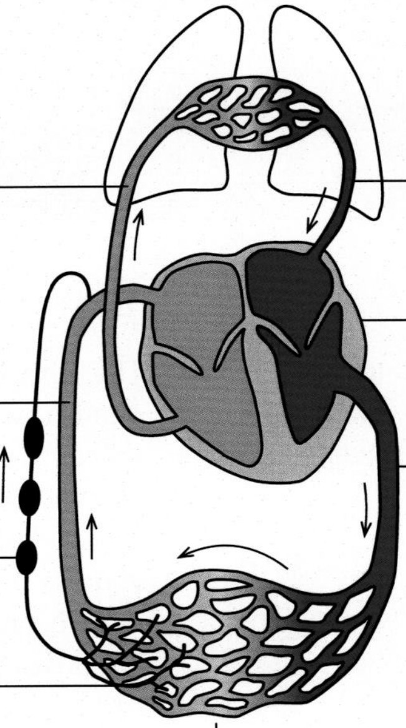
Pulmonary arteries
Pulmonary veins
Heart
Venous system
Aorta-arterial system
Lymph nodes
Lymph vessels
Capillaries

Fig. 1.1 Blood circulation and lymphatic system. [Source: 1.]

blood through the arteries to the capillary bed and through the venous system back into the right side of the heart. In the capillary bed an exchange of substances and movement of fluids between blood and tissue take place. Unlike blood vessels, lymph vessels transport the lymph primarily through a self-activated pumping motion (see section 3.2); the lymphatic system has no central pump.

- **No unobstructed motion through the vessels:** All along the large lymph vessels, lymph nodes are interposed as "filter stations" (see section 1.2).

NOTE

There are also similarities between the lymph and blood vessel systems. For example, lymph transport is fostered by the same factors that favor venous flow. Respiratory motion, arterial pulse waves, and muscle and joint pumps work both on the veins and on the lymph vessels and might also be positively influenced through physiotherapy.

❷ The lymphatic system can be subdivided into four sections. These are distinguished by the size and function of the vessels. The **lymph capillaries** serve to drain the interstitial fluid (lymph formation). **Collectors** and **lymph trunks** are active transport vessels. **Precollectors,** considered from a functional perspective, take a middle position between the capillaries and the collectors.

Lymph Capillaries (Initial Lymph Vessels)
(See Fig. 3.2A)

Between the blood capillaries and the lymph capillaries are the so-called prelymphatic channels. The fluid of the initial lymph vessels flows into these connective tissue channels.

The lymph capillaries form a fine mesh, which covers the body like a net of valveless vessels. In the loose connective tissue of the skin and the mucous membranes, the lymph capillaries lie close to the blood capillaries.

Lymph capillaries have no valves, so the lymph flows in all directions and therefore, in the framework of a therapeutic treatment, can be shifted in a desired direction. Whereas the ciliary arteries of the blood circulation system are often so fine that a red blood corpuscle can pass through it only with difficulty, the diameter of the lymph capillaries is much bigger.

Lymph capillaries consist of endothelial cells, a basal membrane, and attached anchor filaments. The overlapping of the endothelial cells (so-called flap valves) permits the influx of interstitial fluid, which causes the formation of lymph. The lymph capillaries begin with finger-like protrusions in the tissue and can open and shut depending on the need for interstitial fluid (see section 3.1).

Chief characteristics of lymph capillaries:
- Cover the body like a net of valveless vessels
- Have no valves inside the vessels
- Are larger in diameter than blood capillaries
- Consist of endothelial cells, a basal membrane, and so-called anchor filaments
- Have flap valves that enable the inflow of interstitial fluid (lymph formation)
- Begin with finger-like protrusions in the tissue

NOTE

❸ Because of the free movement of the lymph in the capillary net, the therapist can use manual lymph drainage to shift excess fluid in a desired direction for therapeutic aims.

Therapy

After surgical removal of the inguinal lymph nodes, lymphedema of the legs, the outer genitals, and the associated part of the trunk may occur. With drainage strokes the edema fluid can be diverted into the prelymphatic channel and the valveless capillary net in the contiguous regions (see section 6.2).

Precollectors act somewhat like capillaries and somewhat like collectors.

Precollectors

The precollectors are connected to the lymph capillaries and function somewhat like capillaries and somewhat like collectors. Like lymph capillaries, the precollectors have sections in which interstitial fluid is reabsorbed. They also transport lymph to the collectors. In many sections of the wall are isolated smooth muscle cells and valves (see section 3.2).

Collectors

The collectors are the actual lymph transport vessels and have a diameter of about 0.1 to 2 mm. Like venous vessels, they have valves internal to the vessels. The collectors' wall structure resembles that of the veins:

- **Tunica intima** (inner covering) composed of endothelial cells and a basal membrane
- **Tunica media** (middle covering) composed of smooth muscle cells
- **Tunica externa** or **tunica adventitia** (outer covering) composed of elastic fibrous connective tissue

The valves of the collectors are primarily arranged in pairs and have a purely passive function. They prevent backflow of the lymph and guarantee a centrally directed lymph flow (see Fig. 3.4). The distance between two valves is approximately three to ten times the diameter of the vessel. Thus a valve is to be found every 0.6 to 2 cm in the collectors, as opposed to every 6 to 10 cm in the large thoracic duct (ductus thoracicus) (Fig. 1.2).

The section between two valves is called the **lymphangion**. The lymph is propelled by contractions of this section (see section 3.2).

❹ Depending on the location, one can distinguish superficial, deep, and intestinal collectors:

- The **surface collectors** lie in the subcutaneous fatty tissue and drain the skin and the subcutis. Their drainage areas correspond somewhat to the parallel operation of the cutaneous veins. The individual collectors run in relatively straight lines and are connected to each other by anastomosis of numerous branches. When a collector is blocked, the lymph can easily be detoured to other lymph vessels and a stasis (edema) avoided.
- Most of the **deep** (intrafascial) **collectors** of the extremities and the trunk have a somewhat greater diameter than the

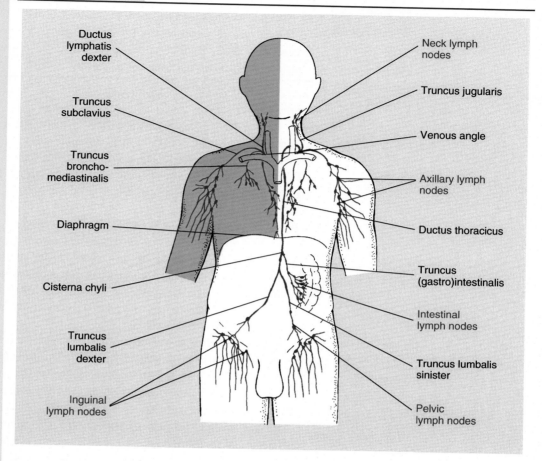

Ductus lymphatis dexter
Truncus subclavius
Truncus broncho-mediastinalis
Diaphragm
Cisterna chyli
Truncus lumbalis dexter
Inguinal lymph nodes

Neck lymph nodes
Truncus jugularis
Venous angle
Axillary lymph nodes
Ductus thoracicus
Truncus (gastro)intestinalis
Intestinal lymph nodes
Truncus lumbalis sinister
Pelvic lymph nodes

Fig. 1.2   The most important lymph trunks of the body and their drainage areas. [Source: 4.]

surface vessels. They drain the relevant muscles, joints, and ligaments. As a rule, they run alongside the deep arteries and veins within a common vessel sheath.

■ For the most part the **intestinal collectors** run parallel to the arteries of the organs to which they pertain.

As in the veins, surface and deep collectors are connected to each other by perforating vessels that penetrate the fascia to make the connection.

Unlike in the veins, the direction of the fluid flow is primarily from below to the surface. Treatment of the surface vessels automatically improves the emptying of the deep vessels (a suction, or so-called water pump effect).

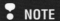

❺ In the arms and legs the collectors essentially run parallel to the extremities and to the joints and are protected in the areas of flexion. In the trunk the collectors follow a star-shaped path to the axillary and inguinal lymph nodes.

Lymph Trunks

The largest lymph vessels are called lymph trunks (trunci lymphatici). These central lymph vessels take the lymph from the inner organs to the extremities and to the sections of the trunk pertaining to them (trunk quadrants). They exit into the venous blood circulation, near the heart.

Lymph Trunks of the Lower Half of the Body

❻ The lymph from the lower extremities and the relevant trunk quadrants, as well as that from most of the pelvic organs, is taken from the **truncus lumbalis dexter** and from the **truncus lumbalis sinister.** These two lumbar lymph trunks join with the **truncus (gastro)intestinalis** and then run to the **ductus thoracicus.**

The ductus thoracicus (thoracic duct), which is about 40 cm long, is the largest lymph trunk of the body. It has a diameter of 2 to 5 mm. Three sections can be distinguished: abdominal, chest, and neck. The intercostal lymph vessels flow into the chest section.

The abdominal section of the ductus thoracicus begins with a sac-like, widened section known as the **cisterna chyli,** which is 3 to 8 cm long and 0.5 to 1.5 cm wide. It lies below the diaphragm (approximately at the level of the first lumbar vertebra) between the rear peritoneum and the vertebral column (see Fig. 1.2).

The truncus (gastro)intestinalis transports the intestinal lymph. The intestinal lymph appears milky after a meal; hence the name "cisterna chyli" for this section of the duct: **chylus** is the milky-cloudy lymph of the small intestine, and **cistern** means "catch basin." The German name, *Milchbrustgang,* comes from this milky cloudiness after a fat-rich meal, as well as its anatomical location.

Lymph Trunks of the Upper Half of the Body

The lymph of the upper half of the body is absorbed on the right and on the left (as the case may be) by three central lymph trunks:

- **Truncus jugularis** (drains the lymph nodes of the head and the neck region)
- **Truncus subclavius** (drains from the axillary lymph nodes, receives the lymph from the upper trunk quadrants, the thoracic gland, and the arm)
- **Truncus bronchomediastinalis** (transports lymph from, among others, the bronchials, the lungs, and the mediastinum)

On the **right** side, the three main lymph trunks come together to form a thick common trunk, the **ductus lymphaticus dexter**. The three lymph trunks of the **left** half of the body flow into the **ductus thoracicus**.

The **vena jugularis interna** and the **vena subclavia** are joined behind the collarbone to the large **vena brachiocephalica**.

❼ The place where the two veins converge is called the **venous angle** (angulus venosus). This is where the ductus lymphaticus dexter and the ductus thoracicus flow into the venous system.

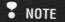 **NOTE**

The **lymph of the lower half** of the body ("everything below the diaphragm"), as well as the **left upper body quadrant**, flows through the ductus thoracicus to the **left venous angle**. The **right upper quadrant** of the body is drained by the ductus lymphaticus dexter into the **right venous angle**.

Practice Questions

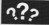

❶ How is the lymphatic system distinguished from the blood vessel system?

❷ Into how many different regions is the lymphatic system divided?

❸ What is the therapeutic significance of the valveless capillary lymph net in the case of edema?

❹ What are the various kinds of collectors, and where are they located? How are they connected to one another?

❺ Explain the path of the collectors to the extremities and to the trunk.

❻ Where do the lymph trunks from the lower half of the body converge?

❼ What is the place called where the lymph trunks flow into the venous bloodstream?

1.2 LYMPH NODES AND LYMPHATIC REGIONS

Human beings have approximately 600 to 700 lymph nodes (nodus lymphaticus [Nl.]; or lymphonodus [Ln.], plural lymphonodi [Lnn.]) with a total weight of about 100 g (4 oz). For the most part they are located in the area of the intestines. However, the head and neck also have many lymph nodes, as do the inguinal and axillary regions.

Structure and Function of Lymph Nodes

Lymph node characteristics:
- A "real" organ with its own blood vessel supply and nerves
- Bean shaped
- 2 to 30 mm long
- Firm connective tissue capsule
- Internal cell network similar to a filter

Lymph nodes function as filter stations.

Lymph nodes are between 2 and 30 mm long and are usually described as bean or kidney shaped. Inside the nodes, which are enclosed by a tight connective tissue capsule, is a fine-mesh network.

❶ It is to the lymph nodes that metabolic waste products, foreign bodies, and pathogens are taken from various cells. The lymph nodes function as filters; they are the cleaning stations of the lymphatic system and occur in groups, or chains of nodes running alongside the blood vessels.

Often the lymph nodes are named for the contiguous blood vessels. For example, the Lnn. iliacales interni et externi (inner and outer pelvic lymph nodes; see section 1.3) get their name from the arteriae iliacae internae et externae (inner and outer pelvic arteries). The name of the lymph nodes simultaneously indicates their position.

Normally, the lymph nodes are not palpable.

❷ Because the lymph nodes are mostly deeply embedded in fatty tissue (e.g., in the axillary area), as a rule they cannot be detected by touch. Enlarged, palpable lymph nodes should always prompt suspicion. Often an inflammation in the drainage area of the node is the cause of the enlargement, although the swelling of a lymph node can also be an indication of a malignant disease. The lymph nodes usually are easily palpable in slim, athletic people. In such cases the fascia of the femur forms a solid underlying layer that prevents the lymph nodes from giving way under pressure. The lymph nodes of the inferior maxillae, usually sensitive to pressure when there are dental problems, may be more palpable in the presence of infection.

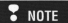 **NOTE**

When lymph nodes are enlarged, the therapist must always consult a physician.

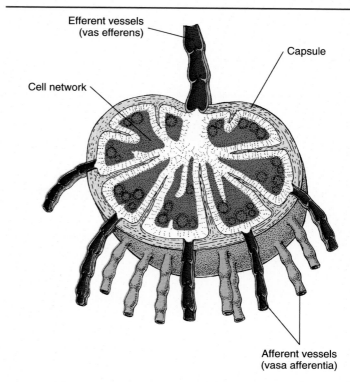

Fig. 1.3 Lymph nodes with efferent and afferent lymph pathways. [Source: 4.]

Lymph nodes have a number of afferent and efferent lymph pathways.

The lymph flows over a number of afferent vessels (vasa afferentia) into the filter-like mesh inside the nodes. At the so-called hilus of the nodes, the efferent vessels (vasa efferentia) exit the lymph nodes (Fig. 1.3). There are fewer efferent than afferent lymph vessels. Also, the overall diameter of the efferent lymph vessels is smaller than that of the afferent lymph vessels. The hilus is the entrance for the lymph nodes into the veins and the arteries.

Lymph Regions

Every lymph node receives lymph from a specific tributary region.

❸ Each lymph node pertains to the lymph of a specific region. This region is called the tributary or catchment region of the lymph node. For example, the axillary lymph nodes are the relevant **regional lymph nodes** for the arm, thymus gland, and upper trunk quadrant. The legs, outer

9

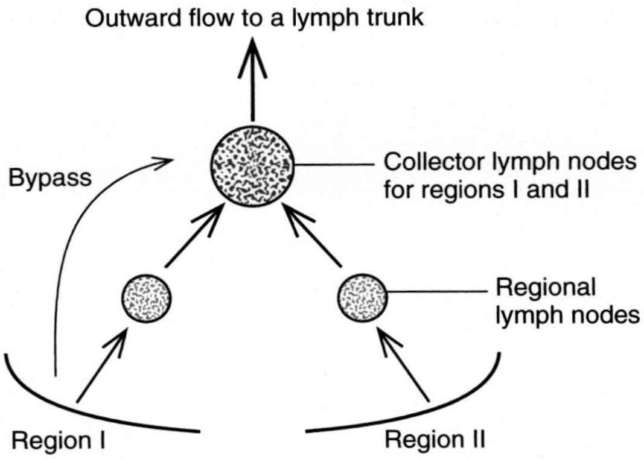

Fig. 1.4 Schematic presentation of the regional division of the lymphatic system by regional and extraregional nodes. [Source: 5.]

genitals, and lower trunk quadrant belong to the tributary region of the inguinal lymph nodes. The lymph from a number of regions flows in extraregional lymph nodes called **collector lymph nodes.**

Finding an enlarged or painful lymph node might lead one to suspect a local inflammation. A painful swelling of the submandibular lymph nodes (Lnn. submandibulares; see section 1.3) might, for example, indicate an abscessed molar.

The lymph nodes play an important role in the spread of cancers. Regional lymph nodes may be invaded (metastasis) by malignant tumors that are located in the tributary region (e.g., breast cancer may metastasize to the axillary lymph nodes). Metastases may occur via regional lymph nodes but may also bypass them. In such a case the cancer goes directly to the contiguous collector lymph nodes (Fig. 1.4).

Although the lymph nodes are defined as individual anatomical groups, it is important to remember that because of their chain-like formation they may also have common functions. For example, the pelvic lymph nodes are regional lymph nodes for the prostate or the uterus. In cases of prostate or uterine cancer, metastases can therefore be found in the pelvic lymph nodes. If these are irradiated or removed during cancer therapy, the result can be lymphedema of the legs, the lower quadrant, or both, since the lymph nodes responsible for this region can no longer transport the lymph to the pelvic lymph nodes.

Germs or metastases from the tributary region can become lodged in a lymph node.

Therapy

The interdependence of the lymph nodes has significance in manual lymph drainage. Treatment of the inguinal lymph nodes is probably not indicated if the person has leg edema caused by surgical removal of the pelvic lymph nodes.

Lymphatic Watershed

❹ The tributary regions of the individual lymph node groups are separated from one another by zones having a scarcity of lymph vessels. These zones are called **lymphatic watersheds.** This metaphor, borrowed from geography, beautifully conveys their function. The collectors of the trunk originate from this watershed like a stream of water from the ridge of a mountain range and flow into other collectors, becoming ever larger.

In the area of the trunk the collectors run radially away from the watershed to the regional lymph nodes, as well as to the inguinal and axillary lymph nodes. The watershed runs horizontally at the level of the navel, as well as at the level of the collarbone; another watershed runs vertically along the body's central axis. Thus the trunk is divided into four territories (two below and two above the navel), called quadrants; in the head and neck area, there are also two quadrants (left and right).

❺ These lymphatic watersheds are not insuperable barriers between the individual trunk quadrants. The valveless lymph capillary net, for example, covers the whole body (see section 1.1) and thus bridges these dividing lines. Moreover, the lymphatic watersheds are bridged by the prelymphatic channel (see section 1.1). These connect blood capillaries to lymph capillaries and run along the connective tissue fibers.

In some locations the large lymph vessels of the trunk wall are connected to the collectors of contiguous territories. The upper trunk quadrants (thorax region), for example, are connected ventrally in the area of the sternum and dorsally between the shoulder blades (interaxillary connections or anastomoses; Fig. 1.5). On the flank, connections exist between the axillary and inguinal drainage areas (axilloinguinal anastomoses).

Therapy

❻ Breast cancer treatment requiring removal of the axillary lymph nodes on the affected side can cause lymphedema

The tributary regions are separated from one another by lymphatic watersheds.

Lymphatic watersheds are not insuperable barriers.

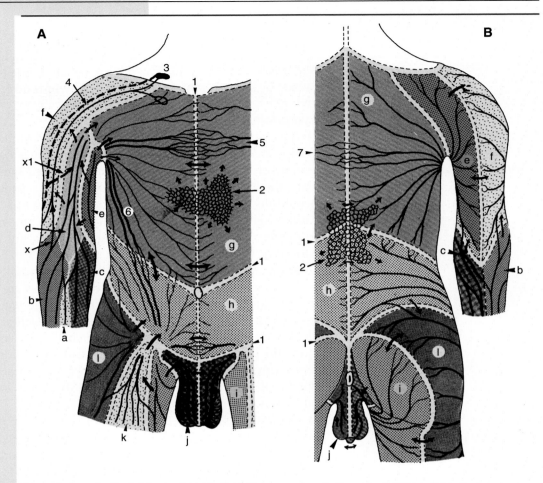

1 Lymphatic watershed at the territorial limits. **2** Cutaneous lymphatic network. **3** Supraclavicular lymph nodes. **4** Lateral upper arm bundle (long: solid line, short: broken line). **5** Ventral intra-axillary anastomotic paths. **6** Axillary-inguinal anastomotic paths. **7** Dorsal interaxillary anastomoses. **a** Middle axillary territory. **b** Radial bundle territory. **c** Ulnar underarm territory. **d** Middle upper arm territory. **e** Dorsomedial upper arm territory. **f** Dorsolateral upper arm territory with deltoid bundle. **g** Upper trunk territory. **h** Lower trunk territory. **i** Dorsomedial femur territory. **j** Territory of the outer genitals and the perineum. **k** Territory of the ventromedial bundle. **l** Dorsolateral upper thigh territory. **x, x1** Anastomotic branches.

Fig. 1.5   Ventral **(A)** and dorsal **(B)** skin territories of the trunk with the adjacent regions of the extremities. Arrows mark the possible drainage tissue after lymphadenectomy.

in the relevant arm and trunk quadrant. The accumulated lymph obligatory loads (see section 2.1) might then be transported by manual lymph drainage either via the capillary net and the prelymphatic channels or via the connecting vessels and anastomoses to contiguous regions with intact lymph nodes. In our example, these would be the territories of the axillary lymph nodes of the opposite side and the inguinal lymph nodes of the same side.

Practice Questions

❶ What are the functions of the lymph nodes? How many lymph nodes does a person have, and how big are they?
❷ Why are most lymph nodes normally not palpable?
❸ What does tributary region mean, and what does regional lymph node mean?
❹ What is a "lymphatic watershed"?
❺ How can the lymph overcome the dividing lines between the tributary regions?
❻ Why is treatment of the inguinal lymph nodes not indicated if the patient has lymphedema of the leg caused by surgical removal of the pelvic lymph nodes?

❖ Practice Section

a) Point out the lymphatic watershed on your partner, and mark the relevant territories and regional lymph nodes.
b) Point out the place on your partner where the collectors run into the trunk area.

1.3 IMPORTANT LYMPH NODE GROUPS AND THEIR TRIBUTARY REGIONS (Fig. 1.6)

Lymph nodes	Tributary region
Lnn. axillares Axillary lymph nodes (can be divided further into subgroups)	Arm and pectoral girdle, upper trunk quadrant (skin, chest muscle), thoracic gland
Lnn. cubitales Elbow lymph nodes	Skin above ulnar part of hand and underarm; wrist, ligaments, bone, and underarm muscles
Lnn. parasternales	Medial section of the thorax, thoracic wall, and upper parts of front abdominal wall, pleura
Lnn. submentales Lymph nodes lying under chin	Chin and lower lip (middle section), tip of tongue and mucous membrane at front section of lower mouth, lower incisors, and contiguous gums
Lnn. submandibulares Lymph nodes lying under lower maxillary	Rest of teeth and gums, tongue, floor of mouth, relevant salivary glands, and palate; skin and mucous membrane of lips and cheeks; nose, tear ducts, middle third of upper eyelid, and conjunctival membrane
Lnn. occipitales Occipital lymph nodes	Back of head and upper part of the neck; neck muscles (might also swell up with inflammation of pharyngeal tonsils)

Lymph nodes	Tributary region
Lnn. retroauriculares Lymph nodes lying behind ear	Rear plane of ear muscle, skin, or mastoid apophysis (in part, also the cellulae mastoideae); skin of head in crown region
Lnn. preauriculares Lymph nodes lying in front of ear	Front plane of ear muscle, skin, forehead, and temple regions; outer part of eyelids and conjunctiva
Lnn. parotidei Parotid gland lymph nodes	Outer ear canal and tympanic recess, parotid gland, connections with Lnn. preauriculares and Lnn. retroauriculares
Lnn. cervicales superiores (laterales et anteriores) Upper (outer and front) cervical lymph nodes	Influx of all head and neck lymph nodes; both surface (Lnn. c. superficiales) and deep (Lnn. c. profundi) Lnn. cervicales
Lnn. supraclaviculares Lnn. cervicales inferior ("Grand Central Station" or "terminus" according to Vodder) Lymph nodes that lie above collarbone or under cervical lymph nodes	Collector lymph nodes for combined neck and head region; shoulder girdle, above collarbone and shoulder blade ridge, cranial part of thoracic gland; thyroid gland, part of trachea and esophagus Metastases from distal organs may traverse connections with the lymph trunks, flow into the venous angle, and settle here; e.g., stomach cancer may metastasize in the left collarbone cavity (Virchow cavity).
Lnn. lumbales Lumbar lymph nodes	Collector lymph nodes of the Lnn. iliacales; scrotum/ovaries, fundus et corpus uteri, kidneys, and suprarenal capsule Outflow over the trunci lumbales to the cisterna chyli
Lnn. iliacales externi et interni Outer and inner pelvic lymph nodes	Lymph from the Lnn. inguinales, urinary bladder. Collector lymph nodes for the organs of the pelvis (prostate, spermatic duct and vesicle, uterus, upper part of vagina—it is not always possible to distinguish the catchment area of the Lnn. iliacales interni from that of the externi)
Lnn. iliacales communes	Collector lymph nodes for the Lnn. iliacales interni et externi; pelvic wall, gluteal muscles, collector lymph nodes for pelvic organs
Lnn. inguinales superficiales Superficial inguinal lymph nodes	Skin and subcutaneous tissue of the lower body (below navel or lower transverse watershed), outer genitals, loins and gluteal region, perineum
Lnn. inguinales profundi Deep inguinal nodes (having a horizontal and a vertical tract in a so-called T-shape)	Lymph from Lnn. inguinales superficiales, muscles, joints, ligaments, fascia and connective tissue of the bones, lymph from Lnn. poplitei; lower third of vagina, uterus, fallopian tube (over round ligament of uterus; lig. teres uteri)
Lnn. poplitei Popliteal lymph nodes	Dorsal and lateral feet and lower shank fascicle, knee region, deep strata of feet and lower shank

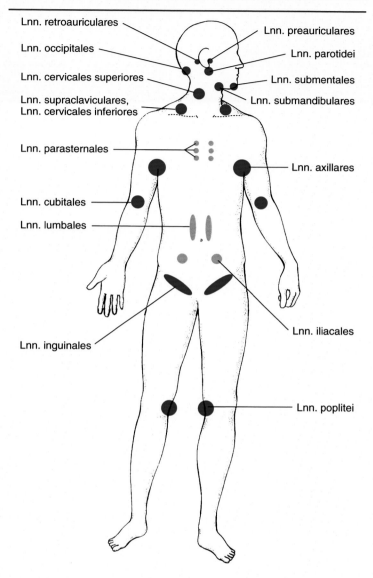

Lnn. retroauriculares
Lnn. occipitales
Lnn. cervicales superiores
Lnn. supraclaviculares,
Lnn. cervicales inferiores
Lnn. parasternales
Lnn. cubitales
Lnn. lumbales
Lnn. inguinales

Lnn. preauriculares
Lnn. parotidei
Lnn. submentales
Lnn. submandibulares
Lnn. axillares
Lnn. iliacales
Lnn. poplitei

Fig. 1.6 The location of the most important lymph node groups.
[Source: 4.]

Lymph is made from
interstitial fluid.

The lymph develops in the lymph capillaries from the interstitial fluid. The interstitial fluid is located in the interstitium (intracell tissue).

2.1 BLOOD AND TISSUE FLUID EXCHANGE

The purpose of blood circulation is fulfilled in the blood capillaries, where the tissues receive nutrients and waste is taken up to be carried away. Fluid is exchanged between blood capillaries and tissue through two distinct mechanisms: diffusion and osmosis. To understand the function and significance of the lymphatic system, one must first be familiar with these two fluid exchange processes.

Diffusion

The wall of the blood capillary is **broadly permeable** to water and to small molecules dissolved in water, such as salt and gases. Because of this it is possible for continuous **concentration equalization** to take place between the blood and tissue. Matter moves from a place of higher concentration to a place of lower concentration. This difference in concentration is called the **concentration gradient.** Through the junctions between the endothelial cells (interendothelial junctions), water, as well as matter dissolved in it, is **diffused** over the entire surface region of the blood capillaries. Fat-soluble substances penetrate the endothelial cells. This diffusion through the blood capillary wall cannot take place completely untrammeled, however. The blood capillary wall is permeable to water and substances dissolved in it, but the passage of individual particles is somewhat hindered because they continually "strike" the walls of the vessel.

By means of **hindered diffusion,** about 240 liters per minute of blood serum containing dissolved molecules flows out of the whole blood capillary system into the

Diffusion: Matter travels along a
concentration gradient through
the blood capillary wall.

16

interstitium. A comparable amount of serum diffuses from the interstitium back into the blood capillaries.

Osmosis and Osmotic Pressure

Osmosis (special case of diffusion): A semipermeable membrane allows the diffusion of water while preventing the diffusion of larger molecules. Through the equalization of concentration, an osmotic pressure arises.

Osmosis can be shown in a container divided in half by a **semipermeable** membrane. Equal volumes of water and aqueous sugar solution are placed in the two sides of the container. The membrane is completely permeable to water molecules, but not to the large sugar molecules. After a certain time the water level increases in the half of the container with the sugar solution. This occurs because the water molecules pass from the part of the container filled with water, where the water concentration is higher, into the part of the container that contains the aqueous sugar solution, where the concentration of water is lower. The sugar molecules, on the other hand, are unable to escape from their section of the container (Fig. 2.1).

Such one-way diffusion, where material exchange can take place in only one direction, is called *osmosis*.

⁕ NOTE

In the osmotic process the sugar molecules had the same effect on the water molecules as a magnet on iron filings.

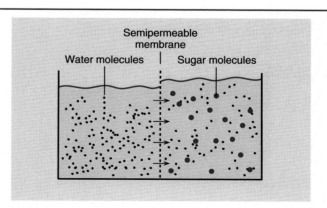

Fig. 2.1   Diffusion of water molecules along a concentration gradient occurring with osmosis. The number of water molecules in the right half of the container increases, causing the water level to rise. Because the large sugar molecules cannot pass through the semipermeable membrane, an equalization of the sugar concentration gradient from right to left cannot take place. [Source: 1.]

Through the increase of fluid, the pressure exerted on the bottom by the aqueous sugar solution is naturally also increased. This pressure, which is determined by the concentration of molecules in the aqueous solution, is called *osmotic pressure*. The more (sugar) molecules that are contained in the solution, the more water that is drawn into the vessel—and the higher the resultant osmotic pressure.

Colloidal Osmosis and Colloidal Osmotic Pressure

❶ About 7 g of protein is contained in 100 ml of blood plasma. The protein molecules are "giants," so-called **macromolecules** or **colloids. Colloidal osmosis** can be demonstrated in a container that is divided by a semipermeable membrane (completely permeable to water molecules but completely impermeable to giant protein molecules). If half of the container is filled with water and the other half with blood plasma, colloidal osmosis will take place. Osmotic pressure, more precisely called **colloidal osmotic pressure,** naturally occurs in the process (Fig. 2.2). Once again, the water molecules pass through the membrane, increasing pressure on the protein side.

Ultrafiltration

❷ By use of mechanical pressure, it is possible to overcome colloidal osmotic pressure. In blood plasma, serum can be

Colloidal osmosis: A semipermeable membrane allows the diffusion of water and prevents the diffusion of giant protein molecules. Colloidal osmotic pressure or suction results.

Ultrafiltration occurs when colloidal osmotic pressure is overcome by mechanical pressure.

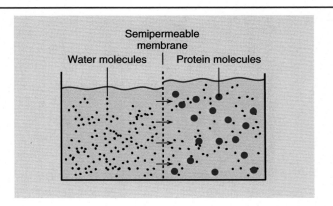

Fig. 2.2 Colloidal osmosis and colloidal osmotic pressure. With colloidal osmosis the behavior of the protein molecules toward the water molecules is similar to that of a magnet on iron filings.

separated from the protein molecules and driven through a semipermeable membrane when the pressure applied is greater than the protein-serum binding force.

An "ultrafilter," a semipermeable membrane, is placed in a pressurized beaker, where the membrane is impermeable to the protein molecule but completely permeable to the blood serum. Blood plasma is placed in the filter. If a piston is used to put mechanical pressure on the blood plasma that is greater than the colloidal osmotic pull of the protein molecules, protein-free serum will pass through the ultrafilter and drip into the flask. This procedure is called **ultrafiltration** (Fig. 2.3). Instead of using a pressure piston, one can create a vacuum in the pressure flask.

NOTE

For ultrafiltration, mechanical forces strong enough to overpower the colloidal osmotic pressure (suction) must be applied.

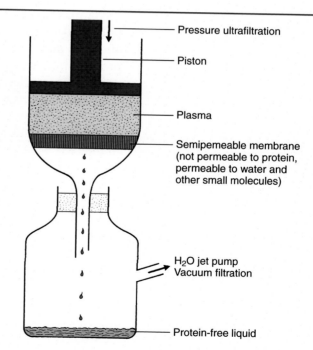

Fig. 2.3   Pressure and vacuum ultrafiltration. [Source: 7.]

The capillary blood pressure (CBP) is the force that drives the ultrafiltrate out of the blood capillaries into the tissue.

Ultrafiltration from the Blood Capillaries into the Interstitium and Reabsorption from the Interstitium into the Blood Capillaries: the Starling Theory

❸ Only the wall of the blood capillaries is permeable to giant protein molecules: some molecules diffuse into the interstitial fluid, and some are found in the ultrafiltrate. In principle, however, the blood capillary wall functions like a **semipermeable ultrafilter membrane.**

The blood capillaries are divided into arterial and venous branches: The arterial branch runs from the beginning of the blood capillary to its middle, and the venous branch runs from its middle to its end. Because the CBP drops continuously from the beginning of the capillaries to their end, the average CBP in the arterial branch is higher than in the venous branch.

The **arterial branch** corresponds to a pressure flask in which the CBP assumes the role of a pressure piston. This overpowers the colloidal osmotic pull of the blood plasma's protein molecule, and an *almost* protein-free fluid is ultrafiltered through the blood capillaries into the interstitium. A complicating factor is that the interstitial pressure (IP) is not equal to zero. If the IP is somewhat greater than zero, and thus positive, this is similar to a situation in which air pressure in a closed pressure flask is slightly greater than the outside atmospheric pressure. If the IP is less than zero, and thus negative, this would correspond to a pressure flask with a pressure below atmospheric. In the former situation, the piston pressure must be somewhat higher than if the pressure in the flask were atmospheric. In the latter, it is sufficient for the piston pressure to be somewhat less than atmospheric pressure to attain the same ultrafiltration. For this reason, ultrafiltration in the arterial branch of the blood capillaries is not the result simply of CBP, but rather of the **effective ultrafiltration pressure** (EUP).

As the IP is subtracted from the CBP, the following calculation can be made:

CBP – IP = effective ultrafiltration pressure

$$EUP = CBP - IP$$

When IP is subatmospheric,

$$EUP = CBP - (-IP)$$
$$= CBP + IP$$

The colloidal osmotic pressure in the interstitium is lower than in the blood.

Because some protein molecules do reach the interstitium through diffusion along with the serum, the interstitial fluid always contains some plasma protein molecules, although the protein concentration of the interstitial fluid is much lower than that of the plasma. This means that a colloidal osmotic pressure (COP_p) exists not only in the blood plasma, but also in the interstitial fluid (COP_i), although COP_i is substantially lower.

Reabsorption: the reentry of fluid into the blood capillaries; fluid is reabsorbed in the venous capillary branch.

COP_p strives to keep water in the blood capillaries and to pull (reabsorb) the interstitial fluid back into the bloodstream. COP_i, on the contrary, holds onto the interstitial fluid and would, if possible, pull more serum out of the capillaries. However, because COP_p is higher than COP_i, the effective reabsorption pressure (ERP) is the victor in this competition, thus maintaining higher COP_p.

$COP_p - COP_i$ = effective reabsorption pressure

$$ERP = COP_p - COP_i$$

❹ Because the CBP is higher in the arterial branch than in the venous branch, the EUP in the arterial branch is also higher than the effective reabsorption pressure: The result is the ultrafiltration described previously. In the venous branch the situation is the opposite; the effective reabsorption pressure is higher than the EUP. Thus the interstitial fluid is pulled back into the capillaries and reabsorbed (Fig. 2.4).

Gross Ultrafiltrate and Net Ultrafiltrate

The gross ultrafiltrate is the combined amount of the fluid ultrafiltrated from the blood.

Some 20 ml/min of serum is ultrafiltered through the blood capillary network as a whole. This quantity of fluid is called **gross ultrafiltrate.** Ultrafiltration and reabsorption do not entirely cancel each other out; only about 90% of the gross ultrafiltrate is reabsorbed. Therefore the **Starling equilibrium** is not perfect.

The net ultrafiltrate is the portion of the ultrafiltered fluid that is not reabsorbed. It is transported out of the tissue via the lymph vessels.

❺ The 10% of the fluid that is ultrafiltered and not reabsorbed is called **net ultrafiltrate.** The net ultrafiltrate is transported away by the lymph vessels and forms the **lymph obligatory water load** (Fig. 2.5).

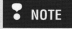 NOTE

The net ultrafiltrate corresponds to the difference between the gross ultrafiltrate and the reabsorbed fluid.

Compared with the diffusion of water at 240,000 ml/min, the volume of ultrafiltrated water, only 20 ml/min, is quite

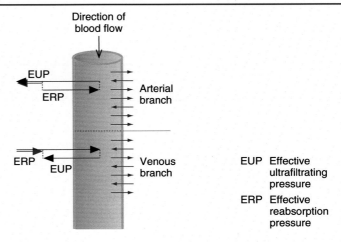

Fig. 2.4   In the arterial branch of the blood capillaries the EUP is higher than the ERP. If the vector representing the ERP is projected onto the one representing the EUP, the resultant vector points outward from the capillary lumen, in the direction of the interstitium: the result is ultrafiltration. In the venous branch the ERP is higher than the EUP. If the vector representing the EUP is projected onto the one that represents the ERP, the resultant vector points from the interstitium in the direction of the capillary lumen: the result is reabsorption. The arrows on the right side of the capillaries symbolize diffusion, which takes place on both sides and in both directions. [Source: 4.]

small. However, the diffusion water is not important for lymph formation and manual lymph drainage. Much more important for manual lymph drainage are the conditions associated with increased production of net ultrafiltrate per unit of time.

For physiotherapists and massage therapists the most significant pathological changes are those associated with an increase in net ultrafiltrate produced per unit of time. This occurs in the following circumstances:

- The effective ultrafiltration pressure (CBP − IP) increases.
- The effective reabsorption pressure (COP_p − COP_i) decreases.
- The effective ultrafiltration pressure (CBP − IP) increases and simultaneously the effective reabsorption pressure (COP_p − COP_i) decreases.

➏ The effective ultrafiltration pressure (CBP − IP) increases when:

The net ultrafiltrate increases when:
- CBP increases
- IP decreases
- COP_i increases
- COP_p decreases

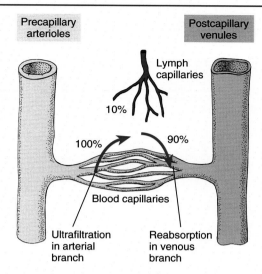

Fig. 2.5 Ultrafiltration and reabsorption in arterial and venous capillary branches. [Source: 4.]

- CBP increases
- IP decreases
- CBP increases and IP decreases at the same time
- ❼ The effective reabsorption pressure decreases when:
- COP_p decreases
- COP_i increases
- COP_p decreases and COP_i increases at the same time
  Corresponding conditions for the increase of net ultrafiltration are the following:
- CBP increases in the case of a **venous obstruction** (passive hyperemia; Fig. 2.6) and with **active hyperemia,** additionally brought about by an acute inflammation and with intense heating of the body through hydrocollator packs or strong massage strokes.
- IP decreases with cachexia (wasting) and with acute inflammation.
- COP_p is lowered with high plasma protein loss through the urine, for example, with some kidney diseases, or through the stool with so-called protein-losing enteropathy. The COP_p also decreases with insufficient plasma protein formation, for example, with certain diseases of the liver.

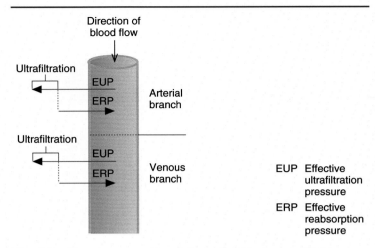

Fig. 2.6 Venous congestion disturbs the Starling equilibrium. Because of the increase in capillary blood pressure that follows passive hyperemia, the EUP is higher than the ERP in the venous branch of the blood capillaries. The result is ultrafiltration in the capillaries as a whole, and reabsorption does not take place. [Source: 4.]

■ COP_i increases with diseases of the lymphatic system, as well as with a pathological increase in the permeability of the terminal vessels to plasma proteins, for example, with acute inflammation (see section 2.2).

It should be noted that the CBP, IP, COP_p and COP_i are **pressures;** net ultrafiltrate, on the other hand, is a **volume per unit of time** (e.g., ml/min). The translation of pressure to volume per unit of time is calculated by multiplication with the so-called capillary filtration coefficients. This means that, besides the previously cited factors, an increase in the capillary filtration coefficients also leads to an increase in the net ultrafiltrate. This is the case, for example, with acute inflammation.

? NOTE

Acute inflammation causes increases in the capillary filtration coefficient, CBP, and permeability of the blood capillaries and postcapillary venules to protein molecules. The COP in the interstitial fluid increases, and the IP decreases. As a consequence, net ultrafiltrate formed per unit of time increases.

Practice Questions

❓❓❓

❶ What does colloidal osmotic pressure mean?
❷ How does capillary blood pressure (CBP) influence ultrafiltration?
❸ Which pressure forces are decisive for reabsorption?
❹ Why is water normally ultrafiltered in the arterial branch and reabsorbed in the venous branch?
❺ What does net ultrafiltrate mean?
❻ What causes the increase in effective ultrafiltration pressure (EUP)?
❼ What processes lead to the lowering of effective reabsorption pressure (ERP)?

2.2 CIRCULATION OF PROTEIN MOLECULES

Efflux of Protein from the Blood Capillaries

The wall of the blood capillaries is not completely impermeable to plasma protein molecules (see section 2.1). Some protein molecules reach the tissue along with the ultrafiltrate. Moreover, protein molecules are continuously leaving the blood circulation through diffusion.

❶ The physiological protein efflux from the blood into the tissue is significant because of the **transport function** of the blood plasma's protein particles: the plasma proteins serve as a means of transport for numerous vitally important substances. These substances are bound to protein molecules and travel with them through the bloodstream to the cells of the body.

❷ In all cases there are substantially fewer plasma proteins in the interstitial fluid than in the blood. That is why the protein molecules are unable to diffuse back into the bloodstream. The diffusion always occurs from where the concentration of molecules is higher to where the concentration is lower. Diffusion can never go "uphill" or against the concentration gradient. To go uphill, molecules need energy (see section 2.1), but there is no gland that can actively draw the plasma protein back into the capillaries.

Return Transport of the Protein Molecule from Tissue

❸ It is important for the protein molecule to exit from the interstitium and get back into the bloodstream. Over the course of 24 hours more than half the protein that is in the

Protein molecules serve as a vehicle for vitally important substances.

The protein molecules cannot diffuse back into the bloodstream.

25

Transporting the protein molecule back into the bloodstream is the most important function of the lymphatic system.

blood leaves the bloodstream. Should these molecules not return to the blood circulation, the consequences would be catastrophic: the plasma protein concentration along with the colloidal osmotic pressure in the blood (COP_p) would drop sharply, and the colloidal osmotic pressure in the interstitial fluid (COP_i) would increase sharply. Simultaneously, throughout the body, there would no longer be any effective reabsorption pressure ($COP_p - COP_i$), and the serum would leave the bloodstream and remain in the interstitium. The result would be **fatal hypovolemic shock.**

Because the plasma protein cannot return to the bloodstream through diffusion, it must be carried back into the blood in some other way. This is the most important task of the lymphatic system.

The lymphatic system takes the protein molecule, along with the net ultrafiltrate and the lymph obligatory water load, and transports them into the venous bloodstream (see section 1.1). Thus the plasma proteins circulate from the bloodstream to the interstitium, from the interstitium to the lymphatic system, and back to the bloodstream (Fig. 2.7) and form the lymph obligatory protein load. Protein hormones injected into tissue by a physician, as well as protein of cellular origin, are also considered part of the lymph obligatory protein load.

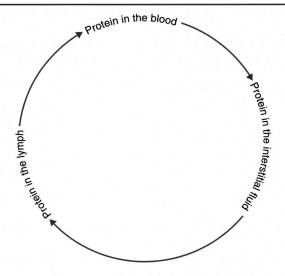

Fig. 2.7 The "extravascular circulation" of protein molecules in blood plasma.

Practice Questions

① Describe the "extravascular circulation" of the blood plasma's protein molecule.

② Why can't the plasma protein return directly into the blood capillaries?

③ Why must the plasma protein be transported back into the blood? What would happen if the plasma protein that leaves the bloodstream were to remain in the interstitium?

Lymph Formation and Lymph Flow: "Physiological Lymph Drainage"

3.1 LYMPH FORMATION

Lymph Formation in Skin Tissue

❶ Lymph is produced in the lymph capillaries through the interstitial fluid that results from net ultrafiltration. The wall construction of the initial lymphatic vessels (Fig. 3.1) is significantly different from that of the blood capillaries; the endothelial cells of the blood capillary wall lie adjacent to each other on a fixed outer basal membrane. Adventitial cells lie on the basal membrane. Between individual endothelial cells are spaces (called pores or junctions) (Fig. 3.1).

In the initial lymphatic vessels, however, the endothelial cells **overlap** like roof tiles. The overlapping parts are movable, hence the name **flap valves.** These overlappings are attached to the interstitium with fine elastic fibers, called **anchor filaments.** The outer sheath of the lymphatic vessel wall

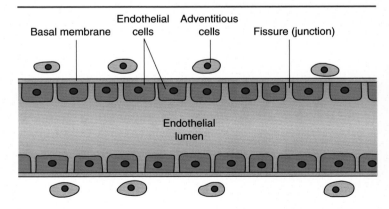

Fig. 3.1 Structure of the blood capillaries: on the inside are the endothelial cells arrayed next to one another, and on the outside a fixed basal membrane and adventitial cells. [Source: 4.]

consists only of loose collagenous fibers. There are no adventitial cells (Fig. 3.2A).

Filling Phase (Fig. 3.2B)
When fluid builds up in the interstitium, the tissue pressure increases and the tissue expands. The anchor filaments are subjected to tension and pull the flap valve up. The junctions between the endothelial cells are transformed into wide-open channels and become "inlet valves." The interstitial fluid flows through these into the initial lymph vessel, in which the pressure is now lower than the tissue pressure. During the filling phase of the initial lymph vessel, the lymph pressure gradually increases. At the end of the filling phase, when the interstitium is emptied, the lymph pressure in the initial lymph vessel is higher than the tissue pressure.

Emptying Phase (Fig. 3.2C)
As long as the tissue pressure is higher than the lymph capillary pressure, the interstitial fluid flows into the lymph capillaries, which lowers the tension in the interstitium.

The flap valves are pulled away from each other.

The composition of the prenodal lymph is different from that of the interstitial fluid.

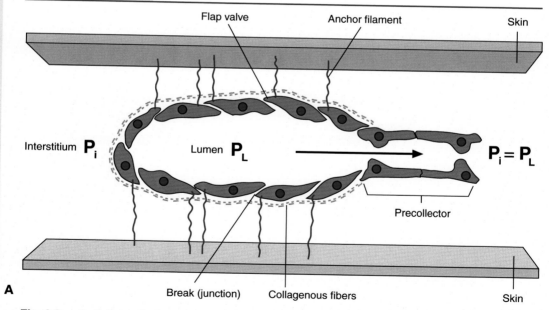

Fig. 3.2 A, Schematic drawing of an initial lymphatic vessel at rest. The inner covering of the wall consists of a layer of endothelial cells with a roof-tile type of overlapping. The anchor filaments are attached to the fibrous scaffolding of the interstitium. The interstitial pressure (P_i) is equal to the lymphatic pressure (P_L). [Source: 4.]

Continued

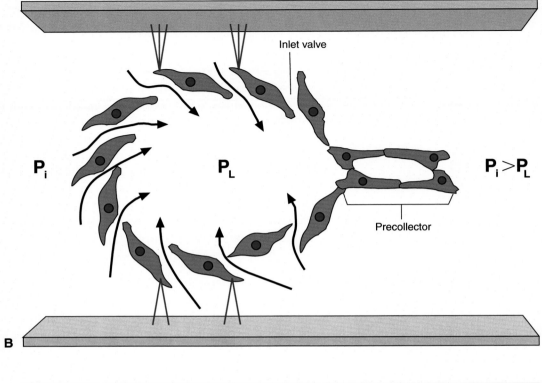

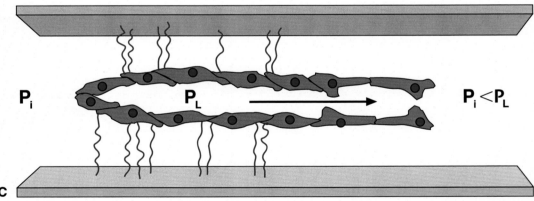

Fig. 3.2, cont'd **B,** Filling phase. The fluid content of the interstitium is increased; the tissue pressure (P_i) increases and becomes higher than the lymph pressure in the lymph capillaries (P_L). The interstitium expands. Because the anchor filaments are fastened to the fibrous scaffolding of the interstitium and to the flap valves of the lymph capillary endothelial cells, the flaps are pulled up, the "inlet valves" are opened, and the lymph capillaries are now closed in the direction of the precollector. The interstitial fluid flows into the lymph capillaries. [Source: 7.]
C, Emptying phase. The fluid content of the interstitium decreases; the tissue pressure (P_i) becomes less than that of the lymph pressure (P_L). The elastic tissue springs back. The inlet valves are closed. The lymph reaches the precollector. One part of the lymphatic fluid is ultra-filtered from the lymph capillaries into the interstitium: the lymph becomes more concentrated than the interstitial fluid. [Source: 7.]

Moreover, the extension of the elastic fibers activates an elastic return force. Just as when a weight is attached to an elastic band that is fixed at one end and then the weight is moved some distance, the elastic will stretch and then abruptly return to its original length, so now the anchor filaments will slacken. As a result, the flap valves are lowered, shutting the inlet valves. The lymphatic pressure is now higher than the interstitial fluid pressure. Now, movement of the body (e.g., a muscle contraction) that exercises pressure on the tissue, or manual lymph drainage strokes of the hand, will suffice to get the lymph to flow out of the lymph capillaries into the precollector. At the same time, part of the lymphatic fluid can leave the lymph capillaries by ultrafiltration and return to the interstitium. Protein molecules, however, are held back. In the process the protein concentration of the lymph becomes higher than that of the interstitial fluid (see section 2.1). Moreover, foreign bodies or pathogens can be captured by the endothelial cells of the lymph capillary walls and phagocytosed (absorbed). The lymph of the afferent lymph vessels (called the prenodal lymph) is thus not identical to the interstitial fluid.

❷ To facilitate lymph formation, repeated pressure changes in the interstitium are necessary. When the body is at rest, not much lymph is formed. Tissue tension, and along with it tissue pressure, must constantly change in order to pump the fluid into the lymph capillaries. Walking, for example, brings about such changes in tension. Manual lymph drainage also effects such periodic changes in pressure.

Lymph Formation in the Muscles

❸ The muscles have embedded precapillary arterioles and initial lymph vessels between bundles of muscles. The anchor filaments of the lymph capillary endothelial cells are connected on one side to the perimysium (connective tissue) and on the other side to the connective tissue of the tunica adventitia of the precapillary arterioles. Because of this structure the systolic vasomotion contracts the precapillary arterioles, leading to the phase in which the lymph capillaries are opened. The diastolic vasomotion, and thus the relaxation of the precapillary arterioles, squeezes the lymph capillaries between the muscle bundles and the blood vessel wall, which brings about the emptying phase of the lymph capillaries (Fig. 3.3).

For improved lymph formation, constantly changing pressure in the interstitium is required.

Systole and diastole of the precapillary arterioles facilitate lymph formation.

31

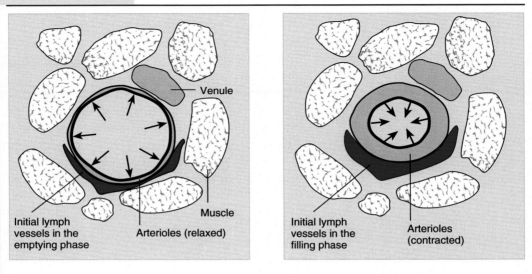

Fig. 3.3 The role of vasomotion in lymph formation in the muscles. During diastole the initial lymph vessels contiguous to the precapillary arterioles are compressed and emptied into the precollector. The systolic vasomotion pushes the lymph vessels apart, so that once again the interstitial fluid can flow into the lymph capillaries. [Source: 3.]

Practice Questions

❶ What is the structure of the lymph capillary wall? What is the structure of the blood capillary wall?

❷ In what way does manual lymph drainage help strengthen lymph formation?

❸ What role do the precapillary arterioles play in lymph formation?

3.2 LYMPH TRANSPORT

Lymph Pump: Lymphangions and the Lymphangiomotor

The lymphangion functions like a little "lymph heart."

❶ The lymph collectors are built from valve segments (see section 1.1) called **lymphangions**. The lymphangions pulsate with an average frequency of 10 per minute. By means of systoles, these **"lymph hearts"** drive the lymph as a pump does (Fig. 3.4). It is possible to obtain a lymphangiogram from a lymphangion.

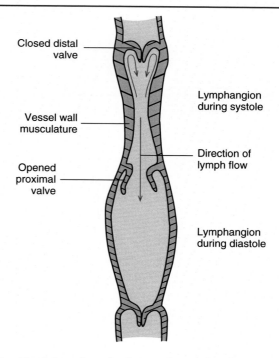

Fig. 3.4   The interaction of valves and vessel wall musculature with lymphangion contraction. [Source: 1.]

NOTE

The lymphangion, like the heart, can carry out its function only if the lymph vessel valves work without any problem. During the lymphangion's systole, the distal valve must be closed and the proximal valve open; during the diastole, the proximal valve must be shut and the distal valve open (Fig. 3.4).

The so-called **lymphangiomotor function** is provided for by the pumping activity of the lymphangion muscles; however, it is also affected by the autonomic nervous system and by various messenger substances. Influences on the central nervous system, such as shock, can likewise change the lymphangiomotor function. This is another way in which the lymphangion functions like a "little heart."

Lymph transport has a special role in subfascial leg lymphatics, where the arteries, veins, and lymph vessels are contained in a common, inelastic sheath. As a result, the pulsation of the arteries acts as a driving force for lymph transport.

Rate of Lymph Output

The Frank-Starling law of the heart states that the cardiac output is governed by the venous backflow.

The lymphangion works, as the heart does, according to the Frank-Starling law. In the heart, this means that the cardiac output is governed by the volume of blood flowing into the right atrium, the so-called preload. If the volume increases by venous backflow, the atrium wall stretches. This strengthens the contraction of the heart muscle so that blood flowing into the atrium is automatically transported further into the aorta. Furthermore, the elongation of the sinoatrial node and the so-called Bainbridge reflex lead to an increase in the pulse.

The lymphangion reacts to an increased inflow of lymph by increasing the rate of lymph output.

The activity of the lymph pump is also governed by the amount of lymph arriving at the lymphangion, the so-called **lymphatic preload.** If the increased lymph output causes an increased volume of lymph, the lymphangion wall and the sinoatrial node within it will become elongated. This causes a more powerful contraction of the lymphangion musculature and an increased pulse rate: the lymph is automatically conducted into the contiguous lymphangion, and the lymph output (i.e., the **volume of lymph per unit of time** flowing into the lymph vessels) increases.

The lymph pump adjusts its activity to the requirements of the organ.

The lymph pump acts not merely by stretching the lymphangion wall, but also by registering the needs of the body at the moment and adjusting the activity of the pump to each situation. For example, when there is a loss of blood, the lymph vessels increase the uptake of interstitial fluid transported into the blood circulation. The lymphatic system counteracts a threatened hypovolemic shock. Through manual lymph drainage massage strokes, it is possible to exercise a stretching simulation on the lymphangions from the outside, thereby stimulating the lymphangiomotor function.

Transport Capacity of the Lymphatic System

❷ The **cardiac output** can increase only when the volume of blood flowing into the veins increases; the preload can increase only up to a certain maximum value. The distinction between the cardiac output at rest and with maximum load on the body is called the functional cardiac reserve.

The transport capacity of the lymphatic system is the greatest amount of lymph that can be transported in a unit of time.

A similar thing is true for the lymph flow rate (LFR): with an increase of the lymphatic preload, the LFR can also rise only to a certain maximum value. This maximum value is called the transport capacity of the lymphatic system. The distinction between the LFR at rest and the transport capacity is called the functional reserve of the lymphatic system.

❸ Only a limited amount of lymph can pass through the lymphatic system in a given time (limited capacity). This lymph output cannot be surpassed even with full activation of the lymphangion motor function.

⏳ NOTE

The transport capacity of the lymphatic system is the greatest possible amount of lymph that can be transported by the lymphatic system per unit of time.

The cell content of the lymph is changed in the lymph nodes.

Role of the Lymph Nodes in Lymph Flow

The lymph nodes not only serve the immune system, but also play an important role in lymph transport.

❹ Under normal conditions a significant portion of lymphatic serum is reabsorbed by the lymph node blood capillaries (see section 1.2). Therefore significantly less lymph leaves the lymph nodes than is transported to them by the afferent vessels. Furthermore, the efferent lymph contains more protein and blood cells than the afferent lymph.

Under pathological conditions, by ultrafiltration, blood serum becomes mixed with the lymph in the lymph nodes. As a result, the efferent lymph output exceeds the afferent, and the efferent lymph contains less protein as well as a smaller number of blood cells than the afferent. This occurs if the lymph nodes are located in an area of venous stagnation or with a subnormal blood plasma protein concentration (hypoproteinemia). Under such conditions the **lymphatic afterload increases,** which can result in afferent lymphatic stagnation. Thus efferent and afferent lymph are distinguished not only by their volume but also by having different amounts of protein and blood cells. In healthy people the efferent lymph contains a greater number of lymphocytes than the afferent, not merely because of the reabsorption of the lymphatic fluid into the lymph nodes, but also because the lymph nodes themselves produce lymphocytes. The afferent lymph contains macrophages that are no longer present in the efferent lymph.

The lymph nodes serve the following nonimmunological functions:

- "Serum reabsorption"
- Lymph reservoirs

Lymph nodes have another nonimmunological function: they can serve temporarily as lymph reservoirs. When the lymph nodes become enlarged by absorbing lymph, the innervated musculature contracts the lymph node capsule through which the lymph is pumped into the efferent lymph vessels.

 NOTE

If the patient has enlarged, palpable lymph nodes, the therapist must inform the physician!

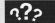 **??**

Practice Questions

❶ What is a lymphangion?
❷ What is the Frank-Starling law for the heart and for the lymph vessels?
❸ What is the transport capacity of the lymphatic system?
❹ What are the nonimmunological functions of the lymph nodes?

3.3 SAFETY VALVE FUNCTION OF THE LYMPHATIC SYSTEM

Section 2.1 described the kinds of change that would increase net ultrafiltrate volume per unit of time and explained that this net ultrafiltrate volume corresponds to the **lymph obligatory preload.** It was further shown that the lymphatic system responds to such an increased preload by increasing the lymph output per unit of time.

❶ The safety valve function occurs when the action of the lymph vessels increases the lymph production per unit of time in response to an increased lymph obligatory water load. Two processes go hand-in-hand with the exercise of the safety valve function. First, more lymph is formed from the increased net ultrafiltrate (corresponds to increased interstitial fluid) in the initial lymph vessels. Second, the lymph pumps are activated by the Frank-Starling mechanism. The lymphangiomotor activity is stimulated.

Were it not for the safety valve function, the interstitial fluid would remain in the interstitium and the tissues would swell. **Extracellular edema** would occur. (An intracellular edema occurs when the cell water content increases.)

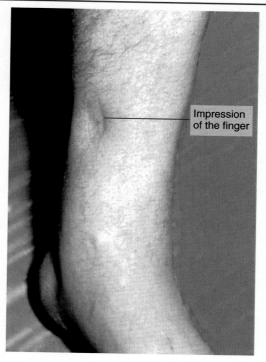

Impression of the finger

Fig. 3.5   Edema in the area of the lower leg. [Source: 8.]

NOTE

❷ **Edema** is called **extracellular** when there is visible and palpable swelling, which is caused by an increased collection of interstitial fluid in the interstitium. Pressing on the swelling with a finger can distinguish such swelling from swelling of the outer tissues: if the swelling is edema, the finger will leave a visible indentation (Fig. 3.5). With **protein-rich edema,** no indentation depression forms because the nature of the edematous tissue changes over time (see section 4.1). This evidence of extracellular edema is not a diagnosis, but merely one symptom.

Practice Questions

?.??

❶ What does safety valve function of the lymphatic system mean?

❷ What is extracellular edema? What is intracellular edema?

4 Lymphatic System Insufficiency

An insufficient lymphatic system cannot handle the required lymph obligatory load and cannot fulfill its safety valve function.

The function of the lymphatic system is to carry away the net ultrafiltrate resulting from physiological rest, as well as to transport the lymph obligatory water load along with the protein molecules dissolved in it, that is, the lymph obligatory protein load. In addition, the lymphatic system is capable of exercising a safety valve function. An inadequate lymphatic system cannot handle the required lymph obligatory load and is unable to perform the safety valve function.

 NOTE

❶ When the lymphatic system is adequate, the transport capacity is greater than the lymph obligatory load. When it is inadequate, the opposite is the case: the lymph obligatory load is greater than the transport capacity.

There are three forms of lymphatic system insufficiency:
- High-volume insufficiency (dynamic insufficiency)
- Low-volume insufficiency (mechanical insufficiency)
- Combined form (safety valve insufficiency)

4.1 HIGH-VOLUME INSUFFICIENCY OR "DYNAMIC INSUFFICIENCY"

High-volume insufficiency:
- Healthy lymph vessels
- Normal transport capacity
- Lymph obligatory load higher than normal transport capacity
- Lymph output corresponding to transport capacity

The lymphatic system can carry only a limited amount of fluid:
- Only a limited amount of lymph can be formed.
- The lymph pump can perform at only a limited level.

❷ High-volume insufficiency (dynamic insufficiency) occurs when the volume of ultrafiltrate produced per unit of time, and thus the lymph obligatory water load that contains protein, is higher than the transport capacity of the anatomically and functionally intact lymphatic system.

❸ Therefore fluid stagnates in the tissue and extracellular edema results. As previously discussed, the reason for this is that lymph output has an upper limit:
- The **lymph formation** cannot be increased without limit (see section 3.1).
- The **lymph pump** cannot increase its output without limit (see section 3.2).

4.2 LOW-VOLUME INSUFFICIENCY OR "MECHANICAL INSUFFICIENCY"

Low-volume insufficiency:
- Diseased lymph vessels
- Reduced transport capacity
- Normal lymph obligatory load
- Lymph output corresponding to reduced transport capacity

- Primary lymphedema
- Secondary lymphedema

❹ Various illnesses of the lymphatic system and lymph nodes can cause the transport capacity to fall below the level of the normal lymph obligatory load, resulting in lymphedema. Lymphedema begins with protein-rich extracellular edema and can lead to heavy tissue damage. It is the most salient indication for complete decongestive therapy, which is an integral component of manual lymph drainage.

Lymphedema occurs in primary and secondary forms. Most **primary lymphedema** is the consequence of a developmental disturbance of the lymph vessels, lymph nodes, or both. **Secondary** forms are caused by various kinds of damage to the lymphatic vessels or the lymph nodes, for example, by malignant tumors, inflammation, lesions, surgery, or radiation.

4.3 SAFETY VALVE INSUFFICIENCY

Safety valve insufficiency:
- Reduced transport capacity
- Increased lymph obligatory load

❺ A safety valve insufficiency arises when the transport capacity of the lymph vessels decreases and simultaneously the lymph obligatory load increases.

Long-term high-volume insufficiency of the lymphatic system can gradually decrease the transport capacity. When the lymphangions work at full power for a long period of time, the pressure in the lymph vessels increases (**lymphatic hypertension**). However, the walls and the valves of the lymph collectors (see section 1.1) are not capable of withstanding this pressure over time. The whole vessel expands under lymph pressure, which may lead to **valve insufficiency.** The valves will no longer shut properly, and during systole of the lymphangions the lymph is no longer pumped solely toward the center, but to the peripheries as well.

Damage to the lymph vessels:
- Lymph node hypertension
- Valve insufficiency
- Wall insufficiency
- Lymphangiosclerosis

If the high pressure in the lymphatic system were to continue, the vessel walls would ultimately become porous, leading to wall insufficiency such that the lymph would ooze through the lymph vessel wall and into the perilymphatic connective tissue. The lymph vessels would become hardened; this condition is called **lymphangiosclerosis.** With low-volume insufficiency, the lymph obligatory load can increase at any time.

39

Consequence of Safety Valve Insufficiency

❻ Safety valve insufficiency leads to combined forms of lymphedema. In the affected areas, cells can die.

Hemodynamic Insufficiency

❼ A special form of safety valve insufficiency, called **hemodynamic insufficiency,** is the consequence of a **right cardiac insufficiency** (Fig. 4.1).

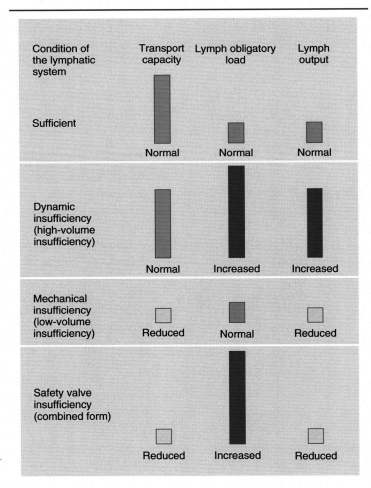

Fig. 4.1   Transport capacity, lymph obligatory load, and lymph output, showing a normally functioning lymphatic system, high-volume insufficiency, low-volume insufficiency, and safety valve insufficiency. [Source: 2.]

Because of inadequate performance of the right cardiac chamber, passive hyperemia is manifested in the blood circulation and the effective ultrafiltration pressure increases.

If the musculature of the right cardiac chamber has been weakened, the chamber can no longer be fully emptied into the lung artery. Blood becomes congested in the right cardiac chamber; this is manifested first in the right atrium and gradually in the venous body circulation as a whole. Venous pressure increases with resulting passive hyperemia throughout the entire blood circulation. The capillary blood pressure rises, causing the effective ultrafiltrating pressure to increase (see section 2.1). Increased net ultrafiltrate is produced, and the lymphatic obligatory preload increases. The lymphatic system reacts with its safety valve function, but this is prevented by the high venous pressure, that is, an increased **lymphatic afterload** that is also present in the left angulus venosus.

If, as a result of the reduced transport capacity caused by the increased afterload, the increased lymph obligatory waterload should exceed the transport capacity, **cardiac edema** (congestive heart failure) will occur.

Practice Questions

❶ What is the relationship between the transport capacity and the lymph obligatory load when there is insufficiency of the lymphatic system?

❷ What does high-volume insufficiency mean?

❸ What are the consequences of high-volume insufficiency?

❹ What does low-volume insufficiency mean? What are the consequences of low-volume insufficiency?

❺ What is safety valve insufficiency?

❻ What are the consequences of safety valve insufficiency?

❼ What does hemodynamic insufficiency mean?

5 Effect of Massage on Lymph Formation and Lymphangiomotor Function

5.1 MANUAL LYMPH DRAINAGE AND LYMPH FORMATION

Manual Lymph Drainage and Lymph Flow Rate

The effect of MLD is an increase in lymph reabsorption.

The lymph flow rate (LFR) can be found experimentally. When the body is at rest, the LFR is very low. If an extremity is subjected to passive motion, the rate increases.

If, besides being subjected to passive motion, the extremity is treated with manual lymph drainage (MLD) **stationary circle strokes** (see section 6.1), the LFR increases.

Increased Lymph Formation

Increased fluid flow into the prelymphatic channels.

The increase in the LFR under the effect of MLD is caused by **increased lymph formation.** MLD effects a stronger pressure, driving the interstitial fluid in the prelymphatic channels of the connective tissue (see section 1.1) into the initial lymph vessels.

Effect of MLD on the Filling and Emptying Phases

The intermittent pressure of MLD accelerates the filling and emptying of the lymph capillaries.

The rhythmic change from compression to extension of the tissue under MLD increases the frequency of the filling and emptying phases of the initial lymph vessels (see section 3.1).

5.2 MANUAL LYMPH DRAINAGE AND LYMPHANGIOMOTOR FUNCTION

MLD fosters the lymphangiomotor function.

Besides its influence on lymph formation, MLD increases the lymphangiomotor function. As a result of increased lymph formation, more lymph is transported to the lymphangion; therefore the lymph vessel wall is pushed outward from within. Furthermore, the stationary circle strokes cause an external dilation of the lymph vessel wall: the Frank-Starling mechanism is activated and the LFR increases (see section 3.2).

As a result of the increased lymph formation and the accelerated lymph transport, the number of lymphocytes transported per unit of time increases.

NOTE

The functional chain of MLD:
- MLD increases lymph formation.
- The increased lymph volume extends the lymphangion wall.
- The vessel wall's stretching leads to an increased lymphangiomotor function (Frank-Starling mechanism).
- The LFR increases.

Practice Question

???

How does manual lymph drainage affect the formation of lymph and the lymphangiomotor function?

6 Basic Principles of Manual Lymph Drainage

Basic Vodder Strokes

The four basic Vodder strokes.

❶ Manual lymph drainage is based on four basic Vodder strokes:

- Stationary circle stroke
- Rotary stroke
- Pump stroke
- Scoop stroke

❷ The motion of these four strokes is based on a common fundamental schema. A distinction is made between the thrust phase and the relaxation phase.

The strokes are subdivided into (Fig. 6.1):

- Thrust phase
- Relaxation phase

The **thrust phase** pushes the fluid in the direction of lymph drainage and acts as a gentle, circular stimulus, promoting relaxation. This stimulation carries over to the lymph vessels of the subcutaneous tissue, which causes an increase in the lymphangiomotor function (see section 3.2). The increase in the interstitial pressure promotes lymph formation.

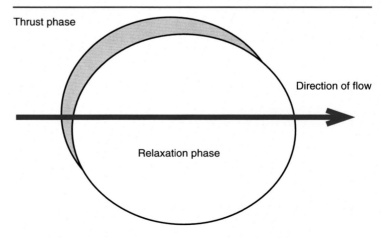

Fig. 6.1   Procedural cycle of the basic strokes. [Source: 5.]

In the **relaxation phase,** during which contact is barely maintained with the skin, the lymph is carried passively out of the tissue so that the vessels can again be filled distally (the so-called suction effect).

The thrust and relaxation phases do not alternate abruptly, but rather go gradually from one to the other and back again. It is important to work at the so-called one-second rhythm, with five to seven repetitions in one place.

NOTE

The basic strokes are adjusted depending on the area of the body being treated. Each stroke is performed five to seven times in one place. The treatment progresses slowly in a distal direction. Three or four strokes returns the flow from distal to proximal at the completion of an area being treated. Throughout the process, the one-second rhythm must be kept with each stroke. As much as possible, the work should be done on the body surface and with relaxed hands.

Edema Strokes

Edema strokes target the free edema fluid to be shifted into the pretreated regions (see section 6.2). The time of thrust is several seconds, during which the intensity of the stroke (see section 6.2) is not essentially increased.

Displacement of free edema fluid through:
- Pump stroke
- Encircling stroke

Two stroke techniques are most commonly applied:
- A two-handed **pump stroke** (the so-called smooth edema stroke)
- An **"encircling stroke"** using both hands; without sliding the hands over the skin, the therapist surrounds the extremity and pushes the edema fluid

These stroke techniques are applied only to the underarms and hands or to the lower legs and feet.

Contraindications

Do not apply edema strokes if the following conditions exist:
- Varicose veins
- Radiogenic damage
- Lipedema
- Pain

Edema strokes must not be applied when patients have the following conditions:
- Varicose veins
- Tissue damage from radiation (radiogenic fibroses)
- Painful lipedema ("fat swellings," i.e., symmetrical adiposus, mostly at the lower extremities; this condition often accompanies lymphedema, and almost all patients are women)

45

Practice Questions

❶ What are the four basic Vodder strokes called?
❷ Into what phases are manual lymph drainage strokes divided?

6.2 PERFORMING MANUAL LYMPH DRAINAGE

Prior Considerations: Resistance to Flow

Because of the high resistance to flow, the strokes must be done slowly and carefully.

❶ When performing manual lymph drainage, the therapist must understand the associated loading of the lymph vessels. The vessels that are affected by the application of the basic strokes have a diameter of less than a millimeter. The vessels of the valveless lymph capillary net (see section 1.1), as well as those of the prelymphatic channel system (see section 1.1), are even smaller. The smaller the diameter of a vessel, the greater the resistance that must be overcome for fluid flow. The hand strokes must therefore always be carried out slowly and gently, so as not to overtax the vessels.

For example, it is easy to quickly empty a full syringe without a needle in it. However, if a thin needle is inserted, making the exit opening smaller, either more force or more time will be necessary to get the fluid out.

Treatment Procedure
Proximal Pretreatment

Each therapy session begins with proximal pretreatment.

Treatment begins with a thorough **proximal pretreatment**. This preparation has crucial significance for the treatment itself.

❷ Through this pretreatment, a proximal area is cleared for the distal edema fluids. As the treatment proceeds, this fluid can be carried away from the stagnant tissue to the area that was pretreated, and from there transported away. Moreover, proximal pretreatment activates the lymphangiomotor function of the proximal lymph vessels for a longer period of time. Therefore a **suction effect** occurs through which the lymph is suctioned away from the distal part (i.e., from an extremity).

The central, healthy lymph vessels that border on the stagnated area might be compared to a conveyor belt. The conveyor belt has to be switched on and running before the fluid of the distal edema is "laid" on it.

NOTE

An extremity should never be treated by simply stroking from distal to proximal without pretreatment!

Therapy

An example of treatment of swelling in the lower leg and foot area:

First the inguinal regions and the upper leg lymph vessels must be pretreated; often pretreatment of the deep abdominal and pelvic lymph trunks is also necessary. Only then can the therapist begin treating the actual stagnant area. Pushing the edema fluid into the pretreated central regions is the last step.

How Firmly Should We Work?

The strokes must be done in a way that achieves the effect without inflicting damage. The hand does not merely slide over the skin. Strokes should be firm enough to stimulate relaxation, but strokes that are too firm must absolutely be avoided.

❸ Too much pressure can damage the thin anchor filaments (see section 3.1). In the area where the collectors are actively pumping, strokes that are too firm might lead to cramps of the lymph vessel wall musculature. On the other hand, work that is too light will not have the desired effect.

Strokes that are too firm might damage the anchor filaments. Strokes that are too light will not have the desired effect.

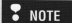 **NOTE**

There is **no generally valid benchmark value for the intensity used** in manual lymph drainage. The stroke must be calibrated to each region of the body. For example, the gluteal region is treated more firmly than the neck. Thus it is not possible to prescribe an optimal treatment pressure.

How Quickly Should We Work?

As mentioned, most work should be done in a one-second rhythm. A faster rate is clearly not indicated because with healthy collectors the frequency of the lymphangiomotor function is no more than approximately 6 pulses per minute when at rest and approximately 20 pulses per minute when in motion.

Working too fast has a negative effect on the ability of the lymph vessels to carry out their function.

Pay attention to position and rest.

What Else Must Be Taken into Consideration?

Increased activity of the lymphangions continues for a certain amount of time after treatment for manual lymph drainage; thus additional time should be scheduled for an after-treatment resting period in a position favoring drainage.

Practice Questions

❶ Why should the strokes be carried out slowly and gently?
❷ Why must the healthy area bordering the stagnated area always be pretreated?
❸ What can happen if strokes are too firm and too rapid?

6.3 INDICATIONS AND CONTRAINDICATIONS OF MANUAL LYMPH DRAINAGE AND COMPLETE DECONGESTIVE THERAPY

Manual lymph drainage and complete decongestive therapy can be successfully applied, particularly with the following diagnoses:

■ Lymphedema (primary and secondary forms)
■ Lipedema (and combined forms such as lipo-lymphedema) and benign symmetrical lipomatosis (Madelung's syndrome)
■ Phlebo-lymphostatic edema
■ Posttraumatic and postoperative edema

The physician who prescribes a certain kind of physical therapy is not always familiar with all aspects of the practical application of the therapy.

This is often the case with manual lymph drainage because, unfortunately, medical studies give little attention to lymphology. Furthermore, over a fairly long treatment, new problems might arise that the physician could not have diagnosed at the time of the prescription.

If the therapist is unsure of anything, the physician must always be consulted.

Various kinds of contraindications:
■ General contraindications for each region of the body
■ Specific contraindications for treating the neck and for pelvic drainage

The therapist must therefore be precisely informed about all the contraindications related to the forms of therapy that he or she employs. If the therapist is unsure of anything, the physician must always be consulted.

A distinction should be made between **general contraindications,** which apply to all parts of the body, and **specific contraindications** in the treatment of the neck and the deep pelvic drainage. Such contraindications are treated separately in the chapters that follow.

A distinction should be made between:
■ Relative contraindications
■ Absolute contraindications

❶ Contraindications can be either absolute or relative. The physician can override relative contraindications if he or she finds good reason, but the absolute contraindications cannot be overridden.

General Contraindications

❷ With decompensated cardiac insufficiency, manual lymph drainage is absolutely contraindicated. This means that cardiac edema (see section 4.3), or congestive heart failure, must not be treated with manual lymph drainage!

Acute inflammation caused by pathogenic germs (bacteria, fungi, viruses) is also an absolute contraindication. The germs could be spread by the manual lymph drainage, with resulting blood poisoning (sepsis). On the other hand, so-called malignant lymphedema caused by active cancer is only relatively contraindicated.

Practice Questions

❶ Can the physician override an absolute contraindication? Explain the difference between absolute and relative contraindications.
❷ Is treating cardiac edema with manual lymph drainage permitted?

6.4 MASSAGE STROKE SEQUENCES FOR DIFFERENT TREATMENT AREAS

The massage stroke sequences presented here, according to E. Vodder, Ph.D., are not to be understood as fixed dogmatic sequences, but rather as sensible aids to learning. The treatment organization is based on the anatomical characteristics of the lymphatic system. It is important to be familiar with, and keep in mind, the ground rules discussed in section 6.2.

The sequence of strokes is determined by the anatomical characteristics of the lymph vessels. The specifics of the stroke technique should also not be considered as dogma, but rather should be adjusted every time to the diagnostic findings. For example, it would not make sense to treat a massive swelling in the area of the foot with the thumbs or fingertips; the flat of the hand would be more effective.

The choice of stroke technique is adjusted based on the diagnosis.

The treatment structure makes up the basis for the treatment of:
- Local disturbances of lymph drainage
- Systemic illnesses with edema

The treatment organization described in the succeeding chapters forms the fundamentals of treatment for the following:

- **Local lymph drainage disturbance:** edema as a consequence of venous stagnation, traumatic and postoperative edema, sympathetic reflex dystrophy (Sudeck's disease), edema accompanied with paralysis
- **Systemic pathological conditions:** diseases whose symptoms include edema, such as diseases in the so-called rheumatism group

Lymphedema, whether primary or secondary (see section 4.2), is always treated with suitably modified stroke techniques and sequences. To pretreat the healthy regions that are contiguous with the stagnated area, the therapist must have mastered the stroke sequences described in later chapters.

Practice Question

Explain the ground rules for performing manual lymph drainage, as discussed in section 6.2.

7

Treatment of the Cervical Lymph Nodes and Their Tributary Regions

7.1 ANATOMICAL FOUNDATIONS

Lymph Node Groups and Territories

The superficial lymph nodes along the neck (lymph nodes [Lnn.] cervicales superficiales) should be distinguished from a deeper layer of cervical lymph nodes (Lnn. cervicales profundi); in addition, the proximal Lnn. cervicales inferiores should be distinguished from the distal Lnn. cervicales superiores (Fig. 7.1).

The lymph of the shoulder and neck region, that is, the upper half of the lymphatic watershed defined by the collarbone and the shoulder blades, drains down toward the lower cervical lymph nodes. Thus the combined lymph of the head and face regions drains to the lower cervical lymph nodes.

Lymph Trunks

Lymph from the head, neck, and face regions reaches the venous system along the:
- Truncus jugularis
- Accessory nodal chain

The lymph of the head, neck, and face regions reaches the venous system by two pathways, where the lymph nodes are linked together like pearls on a chain along the trunk path:
- The truncus jugularis runs on both sides of the vena jugularis.
- The so-called accessory nodal chain (which accompanies the nodus [N.] accessorius) runs dorsally, extending somewhat further, but then likewise flows into the collarbone hollow (Lnn. cervicales inferiores).

Strokes in the neck region must be done as evenly as possible so that both nodal chains may be treated simultaneously.

Therapy

A knowledge of the operation of the lymphatic system helps to save time. For example, in the case of swelling in the lachrymal sac region, it is not necessary to treat the shoulder and neck regions.

51

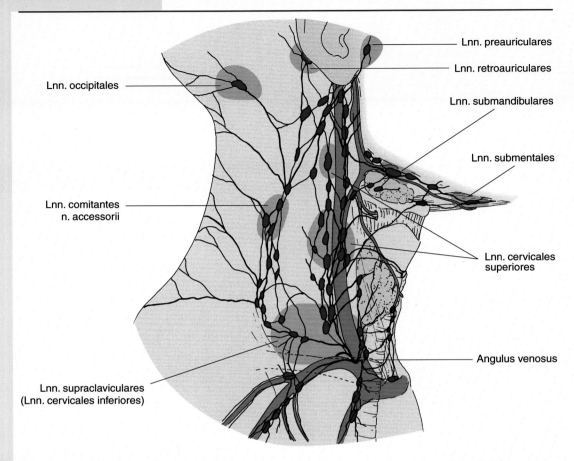

Lnn. preauriculares

Lnn. retroauriculares

Lnn. occipitales

Lnn. submandibulares

Lnn. submentales

Lnn. comitantes
n. accessorii

Lnn. cervicales
superiores

Angulus venosus

Lnn. supraclaviculares
(Lnn. cervicales inferiores)

Fig. 7.1   Anatomy of the head and neck lymph nodes in overview. [Source: 5.] (Modified from von Lanz T, Wachsmuth W, editors: *Praktische anatomie*, vol 1, Berlin, 1955, Springer-Verlag.)

 Practice Section

a) With a partner, find the regional lymph nodes in the head, neck, and face regions, as well as the path of the relevant collectors (see also the illustrations in the following sections).

b) For the following pathological symptoms, consider which regions must be treated and which may be omitted from treatment:
- Whiplash trauma
- Bilateral traumatic edema in the temple and cheek areas
- Edema after extraction of wisdom teeth

7.2 TREATMENT OF THE NECK AND SHOULDER AREAS

Treatment Areas

This section deals with the rear and lateral regions of the neck.

The musculus [M.] sternocleidomastoideus forms the boundary of the treatment area toward the ventral.

Contraindications

Absolute Contraindications

- **Overactive thyroid function,** danger of the thyroid hor-hormones flooding into the blood too rapidly
- **Overly sensitive sinus caroticus,** the threat of a danger-ous decrease in blood pressure and pulse rate (oversensitivity can be the result of a stretching of the lumen at the carotid bifurcation or at the beginning of the arteria carotis interna, where numerous pressure-sensitive nerve endings are present)
- **Cardiac arrhythmia;** in some cases stimulation of the vagus nerve can cause heart failure

Relative Contraindications

Before treating patients over 60 years old, the therapist should consult the referring physician. In older patients, arteriosclerosis in the large neck vessels is always a possibility. The vessels become increasingly sensitive to pressure, and arteriosclerotic deposits might become loosened from the inside wall of the neck arteries and block a blood vessel leading to or actually in the brain (danger of stroke!).

Possible Indications

- Local lymph drainage disturbance after trauma (e.g., whiplash) or after lacerations with formation of significant scar tissue
- Local lymph drainage disturbances after surgery (e.g., dental or jaw surgery)
- Tissue swellings in the area of the head as a result of infections of the ear, nose, and throat region
- **Pretreatment in preparation for further treatment,** treating the Lnn. cervicales inferiores et superiores as well as performing passive motion of the shoulder girdle

---

Margin notes:

- Overactive thyroid function
- Overly sensitive sinus caroticus
- Cardiac arrhythmia

Always discuss older patients with the referring physician.

- Local lymph drainage disturbances after trauma
- Local lymph drainage disturbances after surgery
- Tissue swelling as a result of inflammation
- Pretreatment accompanying other treatments

Stroke sequence for treatment of the neck and shoulder region:
1. Effleurage
2. Passive motion of the shoulder girdle
3. Treatment of the cervical nodal chain
   a. Stationary circles in the collarbone cavity
   b. Stationary circles on the side of the neck
4. Stationary circles on the nape of the neck
5. Stationary circles in front of and behind the ear
6. Stationary circles on the descending part of the M. trapezius
7. Stationary circles on the acromial plateau
8. Finishing work
9. Final effleurage

Preparation
Initial Position
The patient is supine, and the therapist stands by the patient's side.

Massage Stroke Sequence (Fig. 7.2)

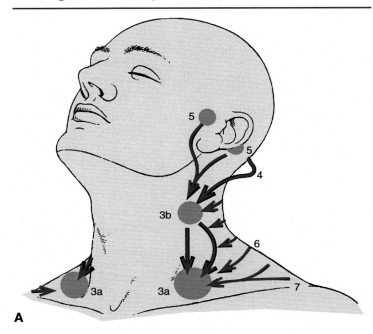

A

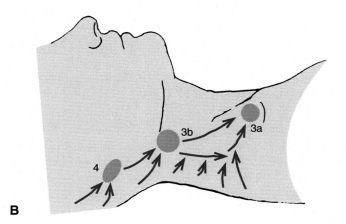

B

Fig. 7.2 Neck treatment in schematic overview. (The numbers correspond to the strokes cited in the text.) [Sources: 1, 5.]

1. **Effleurage**

   Do two or three surface strokes from the sternum in the direction of the acromion.

2. **Passive motion of the shoulder girdle**

   Passive movement, on the one hand, causes an expansion of the large, deep lymphatic trunks (see Fig. 1.1) and, on the other hand, accelerates venous backflow into the vena subclavia.

   The vena subclavia unites with chest muscle fascia, and therefore movement of the shoulder girdle tends to expand the diameter of the vessels (the so-called aeration mechanism). The strengthened venous backflow exercises what is called a "jet pump effect" on the lymph, which is "suctioned" more quickly into the angulus venosus because of the faster-flowing blood.

3. **Treatment of the cervical nodal chain** (Fig. 7.3)

   ■ Carry out **stationary circles** in the collarbone cavity, while in the process doing deep work with light pressure. Vodder calls this treatment of the Lnn. cervicales inferiores a **"terminus treatment"** (Fig. 7.4), because that is where the lymphatic system ends, in the angulus venosus (see section 1.1).

   ■ Finally, using the palms of the hands, apply **stationary circles** on the side of the neck (treatment of the Lnn. cervicales superiores).

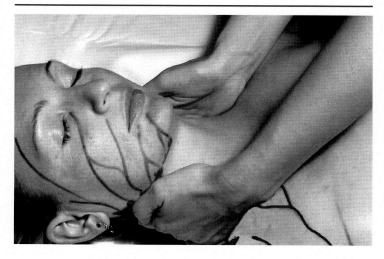

Fig. 7.3 Treatment of the cervical nodal chain. [Source: 5.]

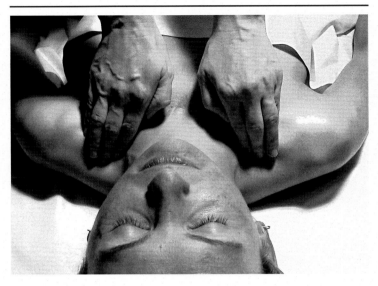

Fig. 7.4 "Terminus treatment." [Source: 5.]

4. **Stationary circles on the nape of the neck**
   - Massage along the linea nuchae (Lnn. occipitales) and from where the spine continues to the spinous process, pushing toward the ventral on the side of the cervical nodal chain (Lnn. cervicales superiores).
   - Finish by draining into the collarbone cavity.
5. **Stationary circles in front of and behind the ear**
   - Treat the Lnn. preauriculares and retroauriculares (Lnn. parotidei) with what Vodder calls the "parotid forked stroke," using the index and middle fingers (Fig. 7.5).
   - Then, drain off through the cervical nodal chain to the collarbone cavity.
6. **Stationary circles on the descending part of the M. trapezius**
   Vodder calls the region above the M. trapezius descendens the "neck triangle."
   - Do stationary circles in the neck triangle.
   - Finally, drain off ventrally into the collarbone cavity. During this stroke the fingertips lie along the spina scapulae, which marks the boundary of the lymphatic watershed (see section 1.2) between the tributary regions of the axillary cavities and the cervical lymph nodes.

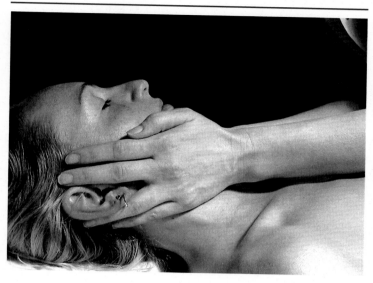

Fig. 7.5   "Parotid forked stroke." [Source: 1.]

7. **Stationary circles on the acromial plateau**
   Move slowly from there toward the medial into the collarbone cavity.
8. **Finishing work**
   This depends on the diagnosis.
9. **Final effleurage**

7.3   TREATMENT OF THE BACK OF THE HEAD AND THE NAPE OF THE NECK

Treatment Area
The spina scapulae (lymphatic watershed; see section 7.1) constitutes the lower border of the treatment area.

Contraindications
See section 6.3.

The general contraindications hold.

- Lymph drainage disturbance after trauma
- Local edema

Possible Indications
- Local posttraumatic lymph drainage disturbances (e.g., after whiplash)
- Local edema (e.g., resulting from injuries)

Preparation
Initial Position
The patient lies face down (prone). The therapist stands beside the patient.

Pretreatment
Neck and shoulder regions

Massage Stroke Sequence (Fig. 7.6)

Sequence of strokes for treating the back of the head and the nape of the neck:
1. Effleurage
2. Finishing work on the cervical nodal chain
3. Stationary circles on the back of the head
4. Stationary circles behind the ear
5. Finishing work on the cervical nodal chain
6. Stationary circles on the neck area, pushing along the cervical nodal chain
7. "Paravertebral treatment"
8. Finishing work
9. Final effleurage

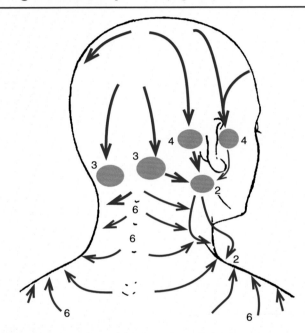

Fig. 7.6 Treatment of the back of the head and the neck in schematic overview. (The numbers denote the strokes cited in the text.) [Source: 5.]

1. **Effleurage**
   Stroke from the back of the head toward the acromion.
2. **Finishing work on the cervical nodal chain**
   Sit or stand at the head of the patient (see section 7.1).
3. **Stationary circles on the back of the head**
   - Do these with the palm of the hand.
   - Begin at the linea nuchae and work up to the "skull area" (called "pyramid" by Vodder). Push in the direction of the Lnn. occipitales or Lnn. retroauriculares.

NOTE The scalp must move along with the strokes.

4. **Stationary circles behind the ear**
   - Do these in the region of the Lnn. retroauriculares (if necessary, also the Lnn. preauriculares).
   - Then drain off toward the Lnn. cervicales superiores.
   - Further drainage follows into the collarbone cavity.

5. **Finishing work on the cervical nodal chain**
   Once again, stand at the side of the patient (see section 7.1).

6. **Stationary circles in the area of the nape of the neck, pushing along the cervical nodal chain**
   - Do **stationary circles** ventrally, from the spinous process toward the cervical nodal chain on the side of the neck.
   - Do **stationary circles** on the M. trapezius descendens ("triangle at the nape of the neck"; see section 7.2, step 6), pushing in a ventral-medial direction toward the collarbone cavity.

7. **"Paravertebral treatment"**
   Do **stationary circles** with the fingertips (called "paravertebral treatment" by Vodder). In the process do deep work with light pressure.

8. **Finishing work**
   This depends on the diagnosis.

9. **Final effleurage**

7.4 TREATMENT OF THE FACE

Contraindications

Infection in the area of the face

Infection in the area of the face (boils etc.) is an **absolute contraindication** for any manual manipulation of this region.

Because the veins of the facial region do not have valves, and given that the venae faciales are connected to the brain via the vena angularis (medially to the eyes), manual lymph drainage might result in the passage of bacteria into the cranial cavity.

Possible Indications

- Posttraumatic lymph drainage disturbance

- Local, posttraumatic lymph drainage disturbances (e.g., lacerations; see section 7.1)

59

■ Postsurgical lymph drainage
  disturbances
■ Tissue swelling resulting from
  chronic inflammation

Massage stroke sequence for
treating the face:
 1. Effleurage
 2. Treatment of the Lnn. sub-
    mandibulares and
    submentales
 3. Stationary circles in the
    lower jaw region
 4. Stationary circles in the
    upper jaw region
 5. Treatment of the nose with
    stationary circles
 6. Treatment of the tear ducts
    with stationary circles
 7. "Long journey" (according
    to Vodder)
 8. Treatment of the upper
    eyelids and eyebrows
 9. Stationary circle from the
    middle of the forehead to
    the temple bone
10. Finishing work
11. Final effleurage

■ Local, postsurgical lymph drainage disturbances (e.g., in
  dental and maxillary area; see section 7.1)
■ Tissue swelling of the head as a consequence of chronic
  inflammation in the ear, nose, and throat region

Preparation
Initial Position
With the patient supine, the therapist sits or stands at the
patient's head.

Pretreatment
Neck

Massage Stroke Sequence (Fig. 7.7)

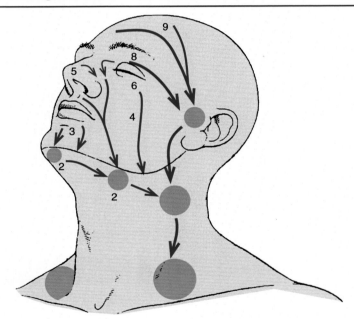

Fig. 7.7   Treatment of the face in schematic overview.
(The numbers denote the strokes cited in the text.) [Source: 5.]

 1. **Effleurage**
    Use parallel strokes over the lower jaw, upper jaw, cheeks,
    and forehead in the direction of the drainage.
 2. **Treatment of the Lnn. submandibulares and submen-
    tales** (Fig. 7.8)

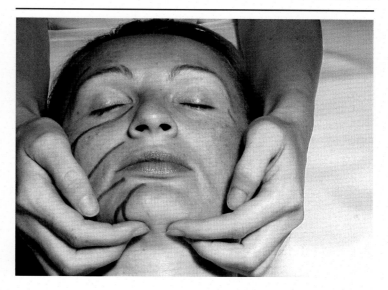

Fig. 7.8 Treatment of the submental and submandibular lymph nodes. [Source: 5.]

- ■ "Hook" the finger under the lower jaw. Pressure is in a lateral direction toward the angle of the jaw and the upper cervical lymph nodes.
- ■ Then drain along the cervical nodal chain into the collarbone cavity.
3. **Stationary circles in the lower jaw region**
   - ■ Treat the chin and cheek areas.
   - ■ To finish, drain off into the collarbone cavity.
4. **Stationary circles in the upper jaw region**
   - ■ Begin under the nose and move toward the cheeks and then to the cervical nodal chain.
   - ■ Then drain off into the collarbone cavity.
5. **Treatment of the nose with stationary circles**
   Stroke with only one finger. Push toward the Lnn. submandibulares.
6. **Treatment of the tear ducts with stationary circles**
   Subsequently, drain off along the Lnn. submandibulares and the cervical nodal chain into the collarbone cavity.
7. **"Long journey"** (according to Vodder)
   - ■ Make stationary circles on the combined cheek and chin regions, pushing toward the Lnn. submandibulares and submentales.

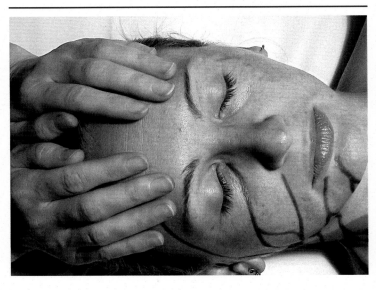

Fig. 7.9   Forehead treatment. [Source: 5.]

- Subsequently, once more treat the Lnn. submandibulares and submentales.
- Finally, once again drain off along the cervical nodal chain into the collarbone cavity.

8. **Treatment of the upper eyelids and eyebrows**
   Push in the direction of the Lnn. preauriculares. Only the inner third of the lymph vessels of the upper eyelid is emptied into the Lnn. submandibulares.

9. **Stationary circles from the middle of the forehead to the temple bone** (Fig. 7.9)
   - Do these with the palms laid flat (Lnn. preauriculares), working in the direction of the angle of the jaw (Lnn. cervicales superiores).
   - Finally, drain into the collarbone cavity.

10. **Finishing work**
    This depends on the diagnosis.

11. **Final effleurage**
    Make parallel strokes running over the lower jaw, upper jaw, cheeks, and forehead.

7.5 ORAL CAVITY DRAINAGE

Infection in the oral cavity

Contraindications

With **infection in the oral cavity,** internal oral drainage is **absolutely contraindicated.** The diagnostic survey must therefore take careful note of inflammations in the oral cavity.

Possible Indications

As a component of the treatment of:

- Primary lymphedema
- Secondary lymphedema
- Tissue swelling with chronic inflammation

- Primary lymphedema in the region of the head
- Secondary head lymphedema (mostly after treatment of malignancies)
- Tissue swelling of the head with chronic inflammation in the ear, nose, and throat region

Preparation

Initial position

The patient lies supine. The therapist stands at the side of the patient.

Pretreatment

Neck, face

Rinse gloves under running water.

The therapist works wearing latex gloves or fingers. Before the treatment these are rinsed in running water to reduce the rubber taste. During treatment the patient is constantly given the opportunity to swallow, and the therapist moistens the working finger with water now and then.

Massage Stroke Sequence (Fig. 7.10)

Massage stroke sequence for oral cavity drainage:

- Cheeks and upper and lower lips
- Hard and soft palate
- Treatment of the mouth floor

1. **Cheeks, upper and lower lips**
   Use **stationary circles** on the mucous membranes of the cheeks and upper and lower lips, offering resistance from the outside.
2. **Hard and soft palate**
   Treat the hard palate and the transition to the softer palate by use of **stationary circles.**
3. **Treatment of the mouth floor**
   Use **stationary circles** on the mouth floor. In the process, exercise counterpressure on the lower jaw.

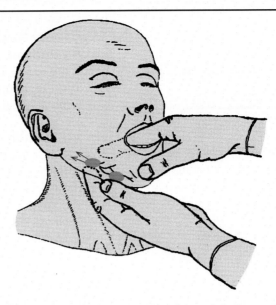

Fig. 7.10   Inner mouth drainage. Treatment of the Lnn. submandibulares with counterpressure from the outside. [Source: 5.]

8 Treatment of the Axillary Lymph Nodes and Their Tributary Territories

8.1 ANATOMICAL FOUNDATIONS

Lymph Node Groups and Territories

The axillary lymph nodes drain the lymph from the arms, parts of the shoulder region, the upper trunk quadrants, and the thymus gland. The axillary nodes can be divided into a number of subgroups. As long as the therapist works extensively with several approaches, all the nodes will be reached during manual lymph drainage treatment; thus knowledge of the subgroups is not crucial.

Lymph Trunks

The efferent lymph vessels of the axillary lymph nodes converge with the arteria [A.] axillaris or A. subclavia and unite at the truncus subclavius.

Therapy

Knowing the anatomy of the lymph vessels can save time. If, for example, the arm is swollen, treatment of the regions of the breast and the back is not necessary. When there is an isolated swelling of the hand (e.g., edema with hemiparesis, traumatic or postoperative edema), the dorsolateral and the dorsomedial areas of the upper arm do not have to be treated.

Practice Section

a) Show on your partner the axillary lymph nodes and the path of the relevant collectors on the arm and on the upper trunk quadrant (Fig. 8.1; see also Fig. 1.5).
b) Consult each other on the following symptoms:
   - Posttraumatic or postoperative swollen shoulder
   - Sympathetic reflex dystrophy (Sudeck's syndrome) of the hand

- Hand swelling with hemiparesis or other paralysis
- Pronounced hematoma on the back of a competitive athlete in your care

Discuss which regions should be treated and which should not. From an anatomical standpoint, what would you consider to be the core treatment area?

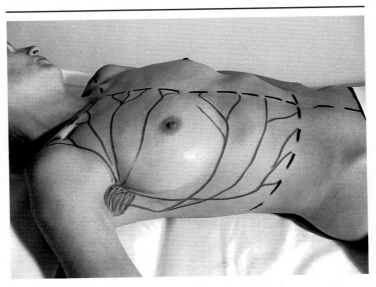

Fig. 8.1 Lymphatic watersheds and schematic presentation of the layout of the lymphatics in the breast area. [Source: 5.]

8.2 TREATMENT OF THE CHEST

Treatment of the upper trunk territory proceeding from the ventral.

Contraindications
See section 6.3.

Possible Indications
As part of pretreatment for secondary lymphedema of the arm (pretreatment of the healthy opposite side).

Preparation
Initial Position
The patient is in a supine position. The therapist stands beside the patient.

The general contraindications hold.

Pretreatment for secondary lymphedema of the arm.

Pretreatment
The neck

Massage Stroke Sequence (Fig. 8.2)

Massage stroke sequence for treatment of the breast:
1. Effleurage
2. Axillary lymph nodes
3. Stationary circles on the flank
4. Stationary circles between the clavicle and the thymus gland (regio infraclavicularis)
5. Treatment of the thymus gland and its lymph vessels
6. Rotary stroke (Vodder's 7th stroke)
7. Finishing work
8. Intercostal and Lnn. parasternales
9. Finishing work
10. Final effleurage

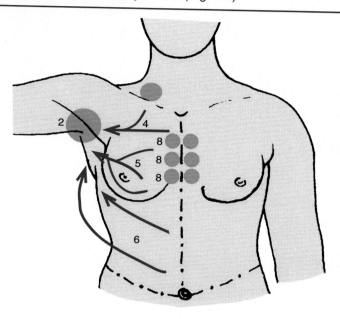

Fig. 8.2 Treatment of the breast in schematic overview. (The numbers denote strokes cited in the test.) [Source: 5.]

1. **Effleurage**
   Make two to three strokes from the sternum to the axilla.
2. **Axillary lymph nodes** (Fig. 8.3)
   Treat with **stationary circles.**
3. **Stationary circles on the flank**
   - Using both hands, begin under the axilla (Lnn. pectorales).
   - Continue to work the horizontal lymphatic watershed at the level of the navel (see section 1.2).
   - Push in the direction of the axilla.
4. **Stationary circles between the clavicle and the thymus gland (regio infraclavicularis)**
   Begin with the sternum, pushing toward the axillary lymph nodes.
5. **Treatment of the thymus gland and its lymph vessels** (Fig. 8.4)

67

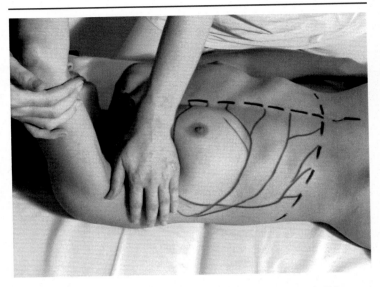

Fig. 8.3   Treatment of the axillary lymph nodes. [Source: 5.]

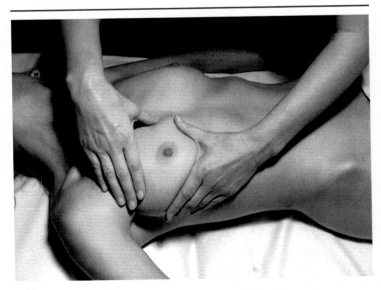

Fig. 8.4   Treatment of the thymus gland. [Source: 5.]

Perform a combination of strokes, consisting of the **pump stroke** (see section 6.1), with the distally located hand, and the **rotary stroke** (see section 6.1) or **stationary circles**, with the proximally located hand. In the process, push in the direction of the axillary lymph nodes.

6. **Rotary stroke (Vodder's 7th stroke;** Fig. 8.5A)
   - Begin under the thymus gland and work over the costal arch toward the flank.
   - Then work with **stationary circles** in the direction of the axilla (Vodder's 7th stroke).

7. **Finishing work**
   - Perform **stationary circles** between the clavicle and the thymus gland (regio infraclavicularis).
   - Work from the sternum toward the axillary lymph nodes.

8. **Intercostal and Lnn. parasternales**
   (For treatment of the parasternum, see Fig. 8.5B.)
   Use springy pressure to work in depth.

9. **Finishing work**
   This depends on the diagnosis.

10. **Final effleurage**

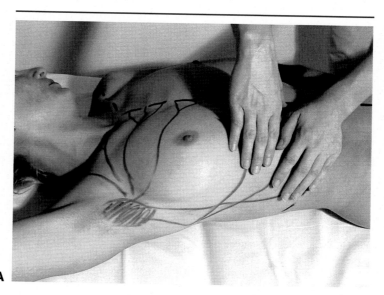

A

Fig. 8.5 **A,** Vodder's 7th stroke on the rib cage. [Source: 5.]

Continued

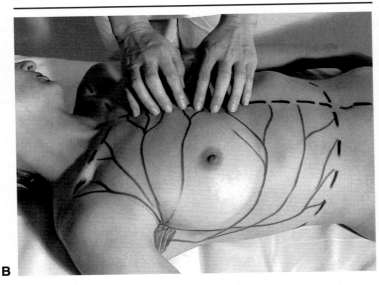

Fig. 8.5, cont'd   **B,** Treatment of the parasternum. [Source: 5.]

8.3   TREATMENT OF THE BACK

Treatment of the upper trunk from the dorsal aspect (Fig. 8.6).

The general contraindications hold.

- Part of the pretreatment of a lymphedema of the arm
- Local lymph drainage disturbance

Contraindications
See section 6.3.

Possible Indications
- As a part of pretreatment for unilateral secondary arm lymphedema (see section 8.1)
- Local lymph drainage disturbances after trauma or surgery

Preparation
Initial Position
The patient lies prone, and the therapist stands at the patient's side.

Pretreatment
Neck, axillary lymph nodes

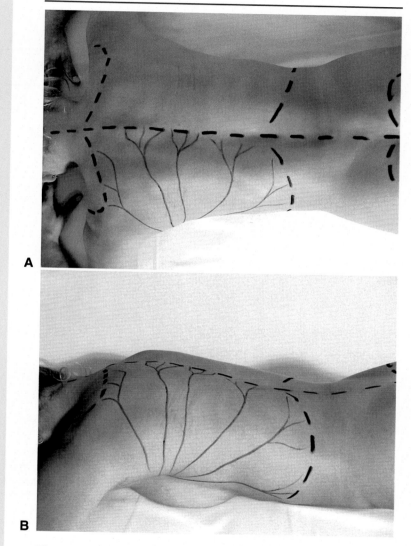

Fig. 8.6 **A,** Lymphatic watersheds. **B,** The large lymphatic paths on the back. [Source: 5.]

Massage Stroke Sequence (Fig. 8.7)

1. **Effleurage**

   Stroke from the extension of the spine in the direction of the axilla.

Massage stroke sequence for treatment of the back:

1. Effleurage
2. Axillary lymph nodes
3. Stationary circles on the flank
4. Stationary circles at the level of the shoulder blades
5. Rotary strokes or stationary circles in the direction of the flank
6. Rotary strokes under the shoulder blade and on the flank (Vodder's 7th stroke)
7. Intercostal and paravertebral treatment
8. Finishing work
9. Final effleurage

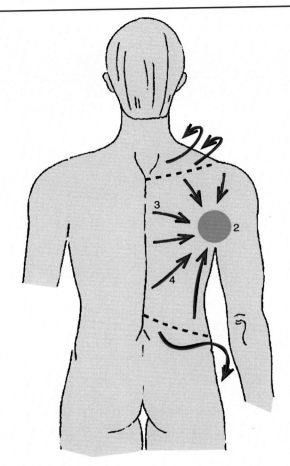

Fig. 8.7 Treatment of the back in schematic overview. (The numbers denote strokes cited in the text.) [Source: 5.]

2. **Axillary lymph nodes**
   Use stationary circles in the axilla.
3. **Stationary circles on the flank**
   ■ Begin with both hands in the axillary region.
   ■ Slowly progress caudally, from the axilla toward the horizontal lymphatic watershed at the level of the navel (see section 1.2).
   ■ The direction of lymph movement is toward the axilla.

4. **Stationary circles at the level of the shoulder blades**
   Using the palms of the hand from the extension of the spine, work toward the axillary lymph nodes.
5. **Rotary strokes or stationary circles in the direction of the flank**
   Alternate from the acantha of the vertebral column in the direction of the flank (medial to lateral).
6. **Rotary strokes under the shoulder blade and on the flank (Vodder's 7th stroke; Fig. 8.8)**
   Alternate (Vodder's 7th stroke) in the direction of the flank; use **stationary circles** to work toward the axilla.

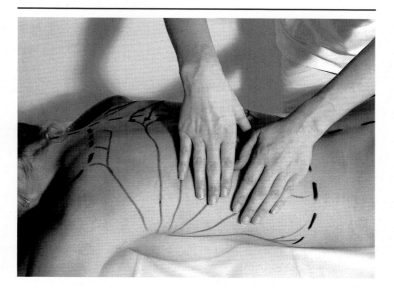

Fig. 8.8   Vodder's 7th stroke on the back. [Source: 5.]

7. **Intercostal and paravertebral treatment** (Fig. 8.9)
   Using **stationary circles,** do deep work with light pressure.
8. **Finishing work**
   This depends on the diagnosis.
9. **Final effleurage**

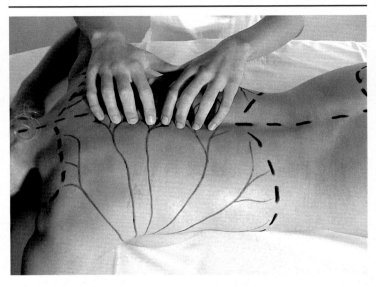

Fig. 8.9   Paravertebral treatment. [Source: 5.]

8.4   TREATMENT OF THE ARM

The general contraindications hold.

■ Sympathetic reflex dystrophy
■ Local edema after trauma or surgery, or local edema with paralysis
■ Auxiliary therapy for rheumatic illnesses

Contraindications
See section 6.3.

Possible Indications
■ Sympathetic reflex dystrophy (Sudeck's syndrome)
■ Local edema after trauma or surgery, as well as edema accompanying paralysis (e.g., hemiplegia)
■ As auxiliary therapy for rheumatic illnesses

Preparation
Initial Position
The patient is supine. The therapist stands beside the patient.

Pretreatment
The neck

Massage Stroke Sequence (Fig. 8.10)
1. **Effleurage**
   Perform in the direction of the drainage.
2. **Treatment of the axillary lymph nodes** (Fig. 8.11)
   Treat with **stationary circles.**

Massage stroke sequence for arm treatment:

1. Effleurage
2. Treatment of the axillary lymph nodes
3. Stationary circles on the inner upper arm
4. Stationary circles on the M. deltoideus
5. Treatment of front and outer upper arm
6. Treatment of the elbow region
7. Treatment of the forearm
8. Treatment of the hand from the dorsal
9. Treatment of the palm of the hand
10. Finishing work
11. Final effleurage

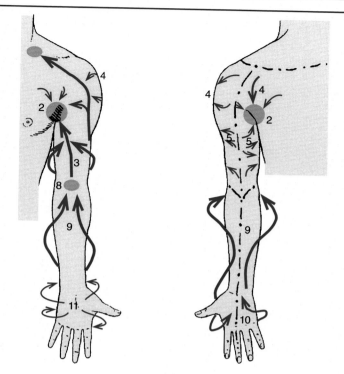

Fig. 8.10 Treatment of the arm in schematic overview. (The numbers denote strokes cited in the text.) [Source: 5.]

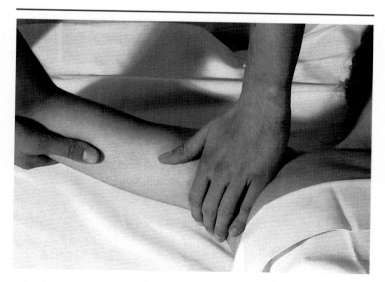

Fig. 8.11 Treatment of the axillary lymph nodes. [Source: 5.]

3. **Stationary circles on the inner upper arm**
   Use both hands on the middle upper arm along the grooves between the musculus [M.] biceps and the M. triceps brachii (sulcus bicipitalis medialis).
4. **Stationary circles on the M. deltoideus**
   Push in the direction of the axilla (Vodder calls this "handwashing").
5. **Front and outer upper arm**
   - Alternate between the dorsomedial and the dorsolateral upper arm bundles.
   - On the upper arm, alternate **pump strokes** with one hand and **stationary circles** with the other hand.
   - Alternate between the front and the outer upper arm (Vodder calls this the "pump and push further").
6. **Treatment of the elbow region**
   - Use **stationary circles** around the inner and outer epicondylus.
   - Push in the proximal direction (Fig. 8.12).
   - Use stationary circles on the elbows (Lnn. cubitales), and combine with passive bending and stretching of the elbow joint.

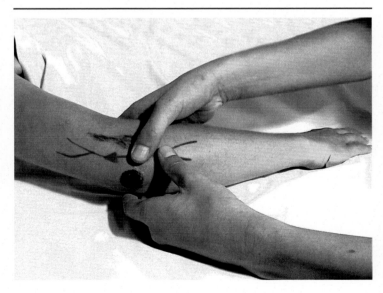

Fig. 8.12 Stationary circles on the medial and lateral of the epicondylus lateralis. [Source: 5.]

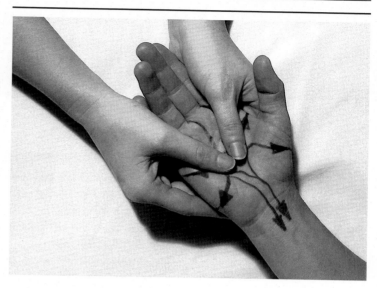

Fig. 8.13 Treatment of the palm of the hand. [Source: 5.]

7. **Treatment of the forearm**
   Use a scoop stroke and **stationary circles** on the flexor and the extensor sides.
8. **Treatment of the hand from the dorsal**
   - Use **stationary circles** on the dorsal along the wrist.
   - Then use **stationary circles** over the back of the hand.
   - Lastly, treat the fingers and the thumb with **stationary circles;** this is done with the thumb laid flat.
9. **Treatment of the palm of the hand**
   See Fig. 8.13.

NOTE

In treatment of the palm of the hand, with exception of the middle ray (middle forearm territory), the inside of the hand must first be drained in the direction of the back of the hand. Only after that should the fluid be driven proximally.

10. **Finishing work**
    This depends on the diagnosis.
11. **Final effleurage**

9 Treatment of the Large, Deep Lymphatic Trunks

9.1 ANATOMICAL FOUNDATIONS

Lymph Node Groups and Lymphatic Trunks

The lymph of the legs, lower trunk quadrant, and genitals flows toward the inguinal lymph nodes.

After passing the inguinal band, the lymph vessels run parallel to the large blood vessels. The lymph nodes are connected like pearls on a chain along the path of the blood vessels. In sequential order:

- Pelvic lymph nodes (outer, inner, and common pelvic lymph nodes)
- Lumbar lymph nodes (often called the aorta cava nodes because they run alongside the aorta and the vena cava inferior)

Because all the lymph vessels of the inguinal lymph node drainage area take this route, a special abdominal treatment is indicated if there is significant swelling in this drainage area.

NOTE

A direct treatment of retroperitoneal structures is obviously not possible. However, by means of special strokes and breathing techniques it is possible to increase the lymph output of these large, deep lymph vessels.

Practice Section

Show on your partner the path and the location of the large pelvic arteries, the aorta, and the cisterna chyli (see section 1.1).

9.2 TREATMENT OF THE ABDOMEN

When a person is breathing in and out, the pressure in the abdominal and chest cavities changes. These changes play an important role in the drainage of lymph from the abdominal and chest cavity organs, the pelvis, and the extremities. This effect is strengthened by deep abdominal drainage that uses special massage strokes and breathing therapy.

Abdominal treatment increases the rate of lymph output through the ductus thoracicus and the other large lymph trunks within the body. This causes a suction effect, so that lymphatic drainage from the legs is also increased.

Contraindications
See section 6.3.

Absolute Contraindications
- Pregnancy
- During menstruation
- Patients suffering from **seizures** (epilepsy), because of the danger of hyperventilation (rapid and deeper breathing), which might trigger seizures
- Blocked intestine (ileus)
- Intestinal diverticulosis
- **Abdominal aortal aneurysm** or after surgical treatment for same
- Massive **arteriosclerotic** changes (mostly in the framework of metabolic disturbances such as diabetes mellitus)
- Diseases involving inflammation of the intestines (colitis ulcerosa, Crohn's disease)
- Pronounced **adhesions in the abdomen** as a consequence of surgical intervention
- Changes in the abdomen or the lower abdominal region after **radiation therapy**
- Radiation cystitis, radiation colitis
- Condition subsequent to pelvic deep venous thrombosis

The general contraindications hold.

- Pregnancy
- Menstruation
- Epilepsy
- Blocked intestine
- Diverticulosis
- Abdominal aortal aneurysm
- Arteriosclerotic changes
- Intestinal inflammation
- Adhesions
- Postradiation changes
- Radiation cystitis, radiation colitis
- Deep venous thrombosis

NOTE

Abdominal drainage must never cause pain. Treatment must therefore always be adjusted to the patient's sensitivity.

- Edema after venous stagnation
- Primary and secondary leg or genital lymphedema
- Secondary arm lymphedema
- Lipedema
- Lymphostatic enteropathy (intestinal lymphedema)

Possible Indications
As adjunct treatment for:

- Edema after venous stagnation (when the relative lymphatics are also affected)
- Primary and secondary leg or genital lymphedema
- Secondary arm lymphedema, especially after double mastectomy
- Lipedema (see section 6.1)
- Lymphostatic enteropathy (intestinal lymphedema)

Preparation
Initial Position
With the patient supine, stand by the patient's side. To relax the abdominal wall, do the following:

- Raise the head of the treatment bench.
- Raise the legs.
- Allow the arms to lie next to the body.

Treatment area
Because the regions of the stomach (epigastrium) and the bladder are particularly sensitive, they are not treated. Furthermore, all work is done along the path of the large intestine to avoid irritation.

NOTE

During treatment, rapid respiration (tachypnea) must not occur.

Pretreatment
The neck

Massage stroke sequence for treatment of the abdomen:
1. Effleurage
2. Modified colon treatment and 7th stroke
3. 7th stroke
4. Intensive, breathing-coordinated strokes
5. Final effleurage

Massage Stroke Sequence (Fig. 9.1A)
1. **Effleurage**
   - During inhalation, move from the pubic bone toward the sternum.
   - During exhalation, move over the costal arch and the iliac crest back toward the pubic bone.
   - Then, with the palm of the hand, use light circles over the solar plexus and the course of the large intestine.
2. **Modified colon treatment and 7th stroke**
   - The caudal hand lies at the descending colon, and the cephalic working hand supports supination motion ("hand-in-hand"). In the process, push toward the cisterna chyli.

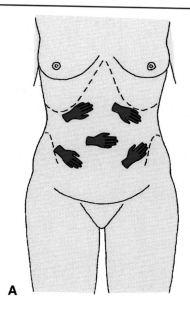

A

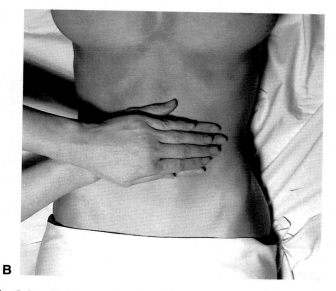

B

Fig. 9.1 **A,** Abdominal drainage in schematic overview.
B, Central stroke. [Source: 5.]

- Next, use hand-in-hand treatment on the ascending colon.
- Along the transverse colon with slightly increased hand pressure, carefully exert firm pressure.

3. **7th stroke**
   - Always work by pushing in the direction of the cisterna chyli.
   - Using increased pressure of the hand, carefully exert firm pressure, slowly moving along the course of the ascending colon.
   - While following the course of the ascending colon, work alternately with the thumb (or the side of the little finger).
   - On the right colon flexure (hepatic flexure), carefully begin to exert firm pressure along the path of the transverse colon.

4. **Intensive, breathing-coordinated strokes**
   These strokes (formerly called "abdominal drainage") are performed at nine different points of the abdominal wall (Fig. 9.1). During this process, remain working at each point for one to three breathing cycles.
   - **Exhalation:** With a light, spirally formed motion in the direction of the cisterna chyli, exert soft but firm pressure.
   - **Inhalation:** Next, exert slight resistance with the hand. As inhalation proceeds, give way and allow the breathing motion to occur freely.

5. **Final effleurage**

9.3 ALTERNATIVE STROKES FOR ABDOMINAL DRAINAGE

Alternative strokes for abdominal drainage:
- Quadratus lumborum strokes
- Respiratory massage

These strokes are used when the traditional abdominal drainage strokes are contraindicated (see section 9.2).

Quadratus Lumborum Strokes (Following Vodder)
- Initial position: The patient is prone. Stand beside the patient.
- Place one or two fingers between the floating ribs and the iliac crest, and pull in the direction of the cisterna chyli.

Respiratory Massage (Fig. 9.2)

- Initial position: The patient is supine. Stand beside the patient.
- Lay both hands on the patient's abdomen, and have him or her consciously breathe with the diaphragm.
- In the inhalation phase, offer a slight resistance (**do not exert deep pressure**).
- Control the breathing by using the so-called pinching stroke on the abdomen.

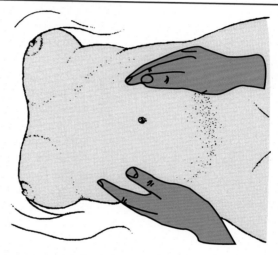

Fig. 9.2   Respiratory massage. [Source: 5.]

10 Treatment of the Inguinal Lymph Nodes and Their Tributary Regions

10.1 ANATOMICAL FOUNDATIONS

Lymph Node Groups and Territories (Fig. 10.1)

A distinction is usually made between superficial and deep groups of inguinal lymph nodes, but for treatment the distinction has no great significance. More important is the division of the inguinal lymph nodes into two major parts forming the so-called **T-shaped inguinal lymph nodes** (Fig. 10.2).

- The upper group runs parallel to the inguinal band (nearly horizontal).
- The lower group, which is located within the femoral triangle (trigonum femorale mediale), runs vertically.

The two groups empty into the same lymphatic pathways that run under the inguinal band to the pelvic lymph nodes.

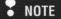 **NOTE**

Attributing a precise drainage territory for these two groups of inguinal lymph nodes is not always possible because the collectors of one area can lead to a number of node groups. Furthermore, the lymph nodes are networked by the lymphatic vessels. Thus extensive treatment over the whole area of these groups of lymph nodes is always necessary.

The **popliteal lymph nodes** empty along the intrafascial lymphatics that run along the vasa femoralia, then drain into the deep inguinal lymph nodes. The superficial inguinal lymph nodes can be palpated, but the popliteal lymph nodes cannot.

Lymphatic Pathways

On the leg it is also possible to distinguish between the superficial and the deep lymphatic system. The deep lymphatic pathways run broadly parallel to the vessel nerve

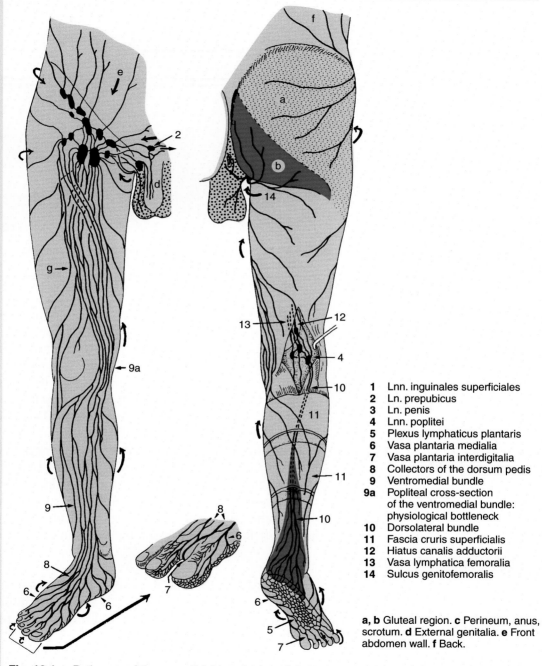

1   Lnn. inguinales superficiales
2   Ln. prepubicus
3   Ln. penis
4   Lnn. poplitei
5   Plexus lymphaticus plantaris
6   Vasa plantaria medialia
7   Vasa plantaria interdigitalia
8   Collectors of the dorsum pedis
9   Ventromedial bundle
9a Popliteal cross-section
    of the ventromedial bundle:
    physiological bottleneck
10 Dorsolateral bundle
11 Fascia cruris superficialis
12 Hiatus canalis adductorii
13 Vasa lymphatica femoralia
14 Sulcus genitofemoralis

a, b Gluteal region. **c** Perineum, anus,
scrotum. **d** External genitalia. **e** Front
abdomen wall. **f** Back.

Fig. 10.1   Pathways of the superficial lymphatics of the leg and the relevant lymph nodes.
[Source: 6.]

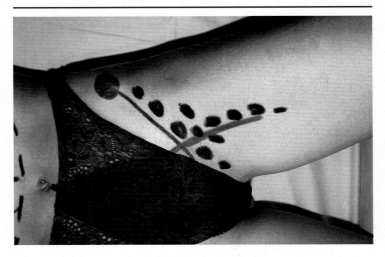

Fig. 10.2 Inguinal region. Diagram of the lymph nodes, the inguinal band, and the arteria femoralis. [Source: 5.]

bundles. Those on the surface run approximately parallel to the two great extrafascial leg veins, the vena saphena magna (ventromedial lymphatic bundle) and the vena saphena parva (dorsolateral lymphatic bundle). The ventromedial bundle begins at the back of the feet and goes up to the inguinal nodes. A bundling of associated lymphatics on the side of the knee (the so-called bottleneck) is of practical significance.

The dorsolateral bundle begins on the side of foot and goes to the popliteal lymph nodes. The lymphatics of the lumbar-buttocks region go to the inguinal lymph nodes. The vessels of the medial side of the buttocks, as well as the perineal region (medial thigh territory), run between the legs to the groin. The vessels of the dorsolateral thigh run along the flanks to the lateral inguinal lymph nodes.

Therapy
Knowledge of the lymph vessel pathways helps save time.
- For a swelling in the lower thigh area, for example, treatment of the lumbar or the abdominal wall region is unnecessary.
- If there is an isolated swelling on the foot, such as after a sprained ankle (so-called inversion trauma), treatment of the dorsomedial and dorsolateral thigh region is unnecessary.

Practice Section

a) On your partner, show the inguinal and popliteal lymph nodes, as well as the pathway of the relevant collectors and watersheds.
b) Consult with each other as to which regions should be treated, and which should not, for the following symptoms:
- Inversion trauma of the ankle, with decided local swelling on the outside of the foot
- Postoperative edema in the knee region following cruciate ligament repair
- Lower thigh and foot edema with chronic venous lymphatic insufficiency

10.2 TREATMENT OF THE INGUINAL LYMPH NODES

Contraindications
See section 6.3.

The general contraindications hold.

Possible Indications
- Component of abdominal wall treatment (see section 10.2) or leg treatment
- Local lymph drainage disturbances after lesions or traumas

- Component of abdominal wall treatment
- Local lymph drainage disturbances

Preparation
Treatment Area
Locate the arteria femoralis to act as a guide. Its pulse beat in the area of the inguinal band serves as orientation for the direction in which to push during inguinal lymph node treatment. A large part of the efferent lymphatics accompany the arteria femoralis and flow into the lacuna vasorum under the inguinal band.

Initial Position
The patient lies supine. The therapist stands at the side of the patient.

 NOTE

When treating the Lnn. inguinales, always work by pushing in the direction of the lacuna vasorum.

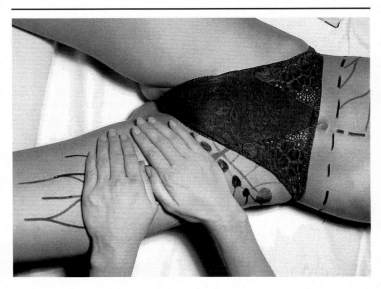

Fig. 10.3   Ventromedial stationary circles in the area of the inguinal lymph nodes. [Source: 5.]

Massage stroke sequence of the inguinal lymph nodes:
1. Laterally
2. Medially
3. Ventromedially

Massage Stroke Sequence
1. **Laterally**
   Make **stationary circles** with the palm of the hand. The hands lie parallel to the leg's longitudinal axis, and the fingertips lie approximately on the inguinal band.
2. **Medially**
   Make **stationary circles** with the palm of the hand. In the process, the thigh is laid slightly abducted and rotated laterally to allow room to work between the legs. The hands lie parallel along the longitudinal axis of the leg, and the fingertips lie approximately on the inguinal band.
3. **Ventromedially**
   Perform **stationary circles** (Fig. 10.3). Both hands lie approximately parallel on the inguinal band, with the palm flat on the trigonum femorale mediale. This also reaches the ventromedial leg lymphatic.

10.3   TREATMENT OF THE ABDOMINAL WALL
(Fig. 10.4)

Treatment of the lower trunk territory from the ventral

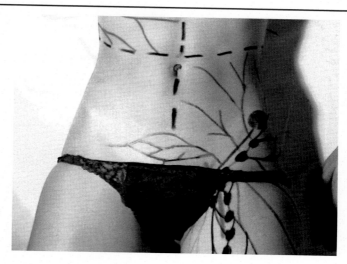

Fig. 10.4   Schematic presentation of the abdominal wall lymphatics, the lymphatic watersheds, the inguinal lymph nodes, the inguinal band, and the arteria femoralis. [Source: 5.]

The general contraindications hold.

- Component of unilateral leg lymphedema treatment
- Local lymph drainage disturbances

Treatment of the abdominal wall:
- Stationary circles on the abdominal wall

Contraindications
See section 6.3.

Possible Indications
- Component of treatment of a unilateral leg lymphedema (pretreatment of the healthy, opposite side)
- Local lymph drainage disturbances after lesions or trauma

Preparation
Initial Position
The patient lies supine. The therapist stands beside the patient.

Pretreatment
Neck, abdominal drainage, inguinal lymph nodes

Massage Stroke Sequence
Perform **stationary circles** on the abdominal wall.
- Use the palms of the hands.
- Use several points of approach, corresponding to the star shape of the surface lymphatics.
- Push in the direction of the lacuna vasorum.

Treatment Area

The lumbar region includes the dorsal part of the lower trunk territory, as well as the buttocks area of the dorso-medial and dorsolateral upper thigh regions (Fig. 10.5).

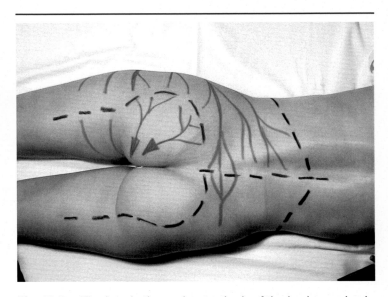

Fig. 10.5   The lymphatics and watersheds of the lumbar region in schematic presentation. [Source: 5.]

The general contraindications hold.

- Lipedema (see section 6.1)
- Component of the treatment of unilateral leg lymphedema
- Local swelling

Contraindications

See section 6.3.

Possible Indications

- Lipedema (see section 6.1)
- Component of the treatment of unilateral leg lymphedema (pretreatment of the healthy, opposite side)
- Local swelling (e.g., posttraumatic)

Preparation

Initial Position

The patient lies prone. The therapist stands beside the patient.

Pretreatment

Neck, deep abdominal drainage, inguinal lymph nodes

Stroke sequence for treating the lumbar region:
1. Effleurage
2. Stationary circles on the flank
3. Rotary strokes on the flank
4. Stationary circles along three pathways
5. Medial upper thigh territory
6. Finishing work
7. Paravertebral treatment
8. Final effleurage

Massage Stroke Sequence

1. **Effleurage**
   Stroke from the sacrum toward the flank.
2. **Stationary circles on the flank**
   Push toward the inguinal lymph nodes.
3. **Rotary strokes on the flank**
   - Work back and forth from the spinous process of the lumbar spine to the flanks (below the level of the navel).
   - From there, push along the pelvic ridge toward the inguinal lymph nodes ("7th stroke" according to Vodder; Fig. 10.6).

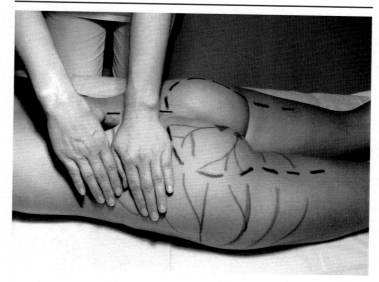

Fig. 10.6   7th stroke in the lumbar region. [Source: 5.]

4. **Stationary circles along three pathways**
   Use **stationary circles** along three pathways, each time with several points of departure (buttocks area lateral to what Vodder calls the "seat of the pants watershed"). Push toward the inguinal lymph nodes.
5. **Medial upper thigh territory**
   Treat buttocks area medial to the "seat of the pants watershed," pushing toward the medial part of the inguinal lymph nodes (Fig. 10.7).

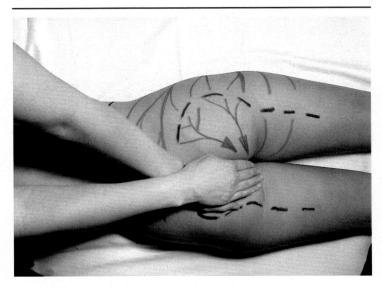

Fig. 10.7 Treatment of the medial part of the buttocks, pushing in the direction of the groin. [Source: 5.]

6. **Finishing work**
   This depends on the diagnosis.
7. **Paravertebral treatment**
   Perform **stationary circles,** firm work with light pressure.
8. **Final effleurage**

10.5 TREATMENT OF THE LEG

Contraindications
See section 6.3.

The general contraindications hold.

Absolute Contraindications
■ Treatment of the leg is contraindicated with **acute vascular conditions.**

■ Acute vascular condition
■ Fungal infection

■ If the patient has a **fungal infection** in the foot, this must be treated first.

Possible Indications
■ Traumatic edema in the region of the foot, often, for example, after inversions or supination trauma ("sprained" ankle)

■ Traumatic edema in the region of the foot
■ Edema with chronic venous stagnation

■ Edema with chronic venous stagnation

Preparation
Initial Position
The patient lies supine. The therapist stands beside the patient.

Pretreatment
Neck, abdominal wall drainage

Massage Stroke Sequence (Fig. 10.8)

Stroke sequence for treating the leg:
1. Effleurage
2. Inguinal lymph node treatment
3. Upper thigh treatment
4. Knee treatment
5. Lower leg treatment
6. Treatment of the foot
7. Finishing work
8. Final effleurage

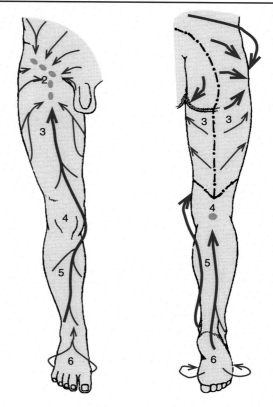

Fig. 10.8 Treatment of the leg in schematic overview. (The numbers denote strokes cited in the text.) [Source: 5.]

1. **Effleurage**
   Work in the drainage direction.
2. **Inguinal lymph node treatment**
   Treatment has three points of departure.
3. **Upper thigh treatment**
   ■ Perform **stationary circles,** also alternating, on the ventromedial bundle (Fig. 10.9).

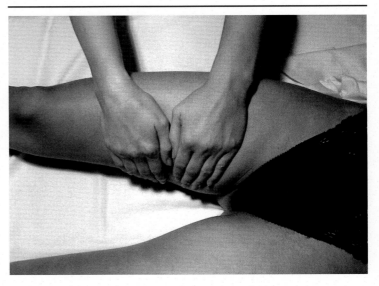

Fig. 10.9 Stationary circles on the inside of the upper thigh.

- Apply **pump strokes,** alternating ventral and ventromedial.
- Use **pump strokes** and **stationary circles** (Vodder's "pump and push along") on the ventral and lateral upper thigh.
- Always push in the direction of the inguinal lymph nodes.

4. **Knee treatment**
   - Apply **pump strokes** over the patella.
   - Treat the popliteal lymph nodes (Lnn. poplitei) with **stationary circles** (Fig. 10.10).
   - Apply **stationary circles** medially to the knee.
   - Apply **stationary circles** running under the pes anserinus.

5. **Lower leg treatment**
   - Raise the leg and use the **scoop stroke** with both hands. If the leg cannot be raised, **stationary circles** can also be used.
   - Perform **scoop strokes** on the calf with one hand; the other hand uses the **pump stroke** over the M. tibialis anterior (Fig. 10.11).
   - Use **stationary circles** under the malleolus and along the Achilles tendon (Fig. 10.12).

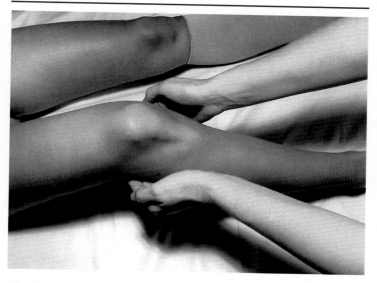

Fig. 10.10   Treatment of the popliteal lymph nodes. [Source: 5.]

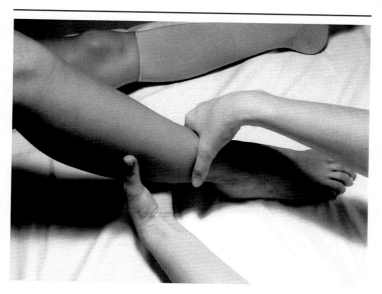

Fig. 10.11   Combination of the pump stroke on the shinbone and the scoop stroke on the calf. [Source: 5.]

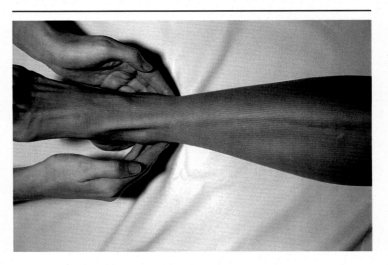

Fig. 10.12 Stationary circles with the fingertips in the region of the retromalleolar grooves. [Source: 5.]

6. **Treatment of the foot**
   - Apply **stationary circles** in the region of the malleolar grooves.
   - Apply **stationary circles** dorsal over the upper ankle (called a "malleolar bottleneck" by Kubik); can also be combined with passive movement.
   - Apply **stationary circles** on the back of the foot.
   - Toe treatment: apply **stationary circles** using the fingertips.
   - Perform an **edema stroke** (see section 6.1) to the front of the foot. The hands encircle the front of the foot, and the edema is very slowly pushed toward the proximal ("lymph sea," according to Vodder).
7. **Finishing work**
   This depends on the diagnosis.
8. **Final effleurage**

Components of CDT:
- MLD
- Compression therapy
- Skin treatment
- Decongestive exercise
- Physiotherapy as required

Phase I:
- Daily MLD
- Daily new compression bandages

Phase II:
- MLD once or twice weekly
- Custom-made compression stocking

11.1 GENERAL

Manual lymph drainage (MLD) is only one component of the **two-phase therapeutic concept** behind complete decongestive therapy (CDT). MLD alone is not a suitable treatment for lymphedema. The following components are at least as important as MLD:

- An accompanying compression therapy (see below for how this functions)
- Therapeutic skin treatment
- Decongestive exercise
- Further physiotherapeutic treatment as required (see below).

During the intensive **Phase I,** treatment is daily and new compression bandages are applied at each treatment. In particular, with advanced forms of lymphedema, this phase is often carried out with the patient stationary. During Phase I, patients also learn how to apply the bandage, which is an important component of the self-treatment measures covered in Phase II. The ability to apply the bandage makes the patient independent and fosters self-reliance.

Within the framework of this book, we discuss only how compression treatment works. A more extensive 4-week course would teach the application of compression bandaging for lymphedema.

Phase II uses custom-made compression stockings (if necessary, complemented by bandages), thus maintaining or even improving on the results of the first therapy phase. In Phase II, MLD does not have to be carried out more than once or twice weekly.

11.2 HOW COMPRESSION THERAPY WORKS

Decrease of Effective Ultrafiltration Pressure

Compression pressure increases the tissue pressure. A disturbed Starling balance is positively influenced because the

97

effective ultrafiltration pressure decreases and so the amount of ultrafiltrate is reduced (Fig. 11.1).

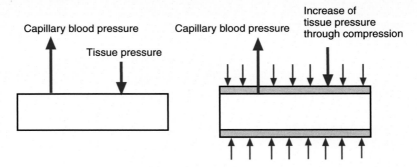

Fig. 11.1   Effects of the bandage pressure on the effective ultrafiltration pressure. [Source: 5.]

Acceleration and Enhancement of the Venous Lymphatic Flow

The narrowing of the vessel lumen leads to an acceleration of flow. The mere use of a compression bandage without any increase in motion will increase the venous speed by 1.5 times, an effect especially important for thrombosis prophylaxis. The lymph output also increases under compression.

The lumen of the dilated vein with insufficient valves becomes narrow, and then the valves again become somewhat adequate. (This mechanism can also be conjectured for enlarged lymph vessels, but thus far this has not been proved; Fig. 11.2.)

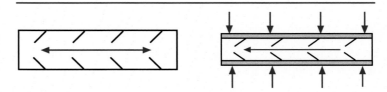

Fig. 11.2   Decrease in the diameter of the lymph vessel under compression. [Source: 5.]

Improvement of the Muscle Pump Function

After the decongestion of an edema, the skin loses its elasticity and becomes slack. Naturally enough, this brings with it an increase in tissue compliance. Only compression bandages (or compression stockings) can give the necessary support to the muscle pumps and increase the efficiency of muscles that foster backflow.

During the calf muscular systole, compression causes an increase in the ejected fraction and a decrease in venous pooling. The pressure drop that accompanies the muscular diastole is intensified; in fact, the pressure in the veins of the calf can even become negative. Because the pressure in the surface (epifascial) veins is now higher, blood is sucked down through the perforant veins, and the overall pressure in the venous system decreases.

The active lymph transport to the collectors (lymphangiomotor function) is also positively influenced.

Preserving Treatment Results

Fluid that has been moved by MLD or by positioning is hindered from backflow. Bandaging preserves treatment results.

Increased Reabsorption Area

Above all, when minor local lymph drainage disturbances (e.g., posttraumatic edema, hematoma) are treated, the edema is distributed over a larger area by the compression and thus the reabsorption surface area is increased.

Increased Elasticity of Fibrotically Transformed Tissue

Compression bandages and insertion of foam pillows can be used to return elasticity to tissue that has hardened as a result of lymphedema (lymphostatic fibrosis).

11.3 DIAGNOSTIC SURVEY

The diagnostic survey, which consists of the case history, examination, and palpation, has several functions:

- It initiates a task-oriented relationship and creates a basis for trust.
- It is a method of concept-oriented gathering and ordering of important data.
- Data processing and synthesis can lead to a conceptual overview, which then becomes the basis for formulating the therapeutic goals and evaluating the treatment results.

The diagnostic survey thus determines the therapeutic plan and the specific therapy to be followed. The clinical picture leading to CDT treatment often includes illnesses seen in internal medicine. For example, lymphedema is often a consequence of cancer therapy.

Because therapists most often treat chronically ill patients over a long period of time, they should know how to recognize, for example, the signs of cardiac insufficiency, acute inflammation, or a recurrence of cancer, and they should consult with the physician when necessary.

The education of physicians obviously cannot include knowledge of all the procedural specifics of MLD treatment. Therefore as a rule the referring physician does not, for example, know that the treatment of the leg requires the treatment of the abdomen or the neck, the contraindications of which must be kept in mind during the process.

The checklist in Fig. 11.3 does not claim to be exhaustive. However, this checklist has proved useful in everyday application and has been very helpful at the beginning of treatment of patients with lymphedema. The conclusions should always be discussed with the aftercare worker, the prescribing physician, or both.

For reasons of space, Fig. 11.3 gives only a general picture of diagnostic surveys, and certain knowledge on the part of the reader is assumed (e.g., palpation should be performed only with warm hands; the patient should be disrobed to the level of his or her comfort for the examination).

11.4 FURTHER PHYSICAL THERAPY MEASURES WITHIN THE CDT FRAMEWORK

Heat Application

Hyperemia always leads to an increase in the lymph obligatory load. For this reason, heat applications, such as hydrocollator packs and mudpacks, are contraindicated in the area of the edema (this includes the relevant trunk quadrants). Moreover, at temperatures above 41° C (105° F), the rate of lymph production decreases.

Our experience has shown that local heat application, except on the edematous areas, does not exacerbate the condition. For example, for a patient with a secondary arm lymphedema after the removal of the axillary lymph nodes, heat application to the thoracic vertebra is contraindicated.

MLD/CDT Diagnostic Survey Checklist

Name

Diagnosis   Intake   by

Prescription   on

Edema-Related Medical History
Surgical history?
Radiation therapy?   Yes ○   No ○
Other postsurgery treatments?
When and how was the edema first manifested? Triggering factors? Erysipelas? Recurrent?
History of development and treatment of the edema?
What kinds of problems give you the **most** trouble at this time?
Subjective: How does the edema feel to the patient?

Edema-Related Diagnostic Findings (see also under diagnostic findings "Body Chart")
Skin changes? Edema consistency – do impressions in the skin remain? Lymphostatic fibrosis?
"Tautness of skin": Is the edema only distal from the knee/elbow? Central accentuation? Skin fold test on trunk quadrant?
"Pure" LE ○   Combined form (varicosis, lipedema, cyclical idiopathic edema syndrome, etc.) ○

Quantitative Measurement   Date   Time   (body weight   kg)

Point 1   Point 3

Point 2   Point 4

Complications Scar tissue, reflux-lymphatic cysts or fistulas? Skin lesions, mycoses, eczema; changes in the nails; signs of inflammation, ulceration, etc.?
Is radiation-induced damage visible or palpable?   Yes ○   No ○
Indications of a malignant process?
Collateral veins? Are there palpable, suspicious nodes (lymph nodes)? Neck-acromion distance?
Accumulation of supraclavicular grooves? Pain, sensory disturbance? Paresis/paralysis?
Changes in the skin? Color changes?

Fig. 11.3   MLD/CDT Diagnostic Survey Checklist. *CDT,* Complete decongestive therapy; *MLD,* manual lymph drainage.

Continued

Overview – Areas of Note				
Head and neck?	Yes ○		No ○	
Chest and back?	Yes ○		No ○	
Thymus gland?	Yes ○		No ○	
Abdomen?	Yes ○		No ○	

Other illnesses? What medications is the patient taking?

For women: short menstrual history

"Body Chart" and Treatment Organization

Edema-Related Procedure (Dimensions[1])

	Date	Date	Date	Date	Date	Date	Date	Date	Date
Point 1									
Point 2									
Point 3									
Point 4									
Weight									
Time of day									

[1] In daily clinical practice, the size of the area afflicted with edema is sufficiently indicated with a few pronounced and reproducible points; more precise measurement of the size and calculation of the volume are required when more scientific questions are involved (the so-called 4 cm disk model). Volume determination using water replacement or photoelectric methods is likewise reserved for scientific questions.

Fig. 11.3, cont'd   MLD/CDT Diagnostic Survey Checklist. *CDT,* Complete decongestive therapy; *MLD,* manual lymph drainage.   *Continued*

Functional Diagnostic Findings

Range of motion in the relevant joints (active and passive)

Examples of motion/Relieving posture/Avoidance of movement/Muscle tone

"Everyday activities": What is possible, what is not? Why not? What causes problems?
Functional deficit? Treatable lack of strength?

Therapy Plan

| Is **pain treatment** required first? | Yes ○ | No ○ |

Decongestive or conservation **phase** necessary? Degree of severity of the edema? "Condition" of the
compression stockings?

| **Self-bandaging** possible? | Yes ○ | No ○ |
| Is the edema patient familiar with the **explanatory brochure?** | Yes ○ | No ○ |

Other therapeutic targets (lack of strength, reduced range of motion, etc.)?

| **Consultation** with physician **necessary?** | Yes ○ | No ○ |

Agreement on Therapeutic Goals

Therapeutic goals to be explained to the patient, preserved in writing, and reviewed at the end of therapy.

Fig. 11.3, cont'd MLD/CDT Diagnostic Survey Checklist. *CDT,* Complete decongestive therapy;
MLD, manual lymph drainage.

Conversely, if the patient has a disorder in the lumbar region without edema, there is no reason to oppose a local heat application.

Whole body heat applications, such as sauna, rising temperature baths, and thermal baths, are contraindicated.

Cooling

Cryotherapy is an established part of sports physiotherapy. However, there should always be an interlude of 20 minutes between cooling and the beginning of therapy. Cold applications are not indicated for treatment of the lymph nodes of the extremities because the cold leads to a reduced lymphangiomotor function.

If indicated (e.g., with sympathetic reflex dystrophy), mild cooling can be followed by a moist pack.

Hydrotherapy

Hydrotherapeutic measures have been shown to be especially useful in therapy for those with venous legs, yet hydrotherapy is not unconditionally indicated for treatment of lymph node edema of the extremities. Swimming is favorable (increased outside pressure) with water temperatures between 22° and 30° C (maximum) (71° and 86° F).

Electrotherapy

Because of extreme tendencies toward hyperemia, and the concomitant increase in the lymph obligatory load, DC current and the hydroelectric bath are contraindicated.

Ultrasound, interference currents, or transcutaneous electrical nerve stimulation (TENS), however, can be applied if indications for them are present.

Massage

Traditional massage and connective tissue massage are contraindicated in the edematous area and thus also in the related trunk quadrants.

However, when the use of Marnitz therapy has been indicated, it has proved very useful.

Index

A

Abdomen, manual lymph drainage of, 79-83
  contraindications to, 79
Abdominal wall, manual lymph drainage of, 88-89
Acromial plateau, stationary circle strokes on, 57
Anastomoses, axilloinguinal, 11
Anchor filaments, of lymph capillaries, 3, 28, 29, 31
Ankle, inversions or supinations of, 86, 87, 92
Arm
  collectors in, 5
  lymphedema of, manual lymph drainage pretreatment
    for, 66, 70
  manual lymph drainage of, 74-77
Arteria femoralis, 86, 87, 89
Arterioles, precapillary, 31, 32
Axillary lymph nodes
  anatomy of, 65-66
  location of, 15
  manual lymph drainage of, 66-77
  surgical removal of, 11-13
  tributary (drainage) regions of, 9-10, 13, 65

B

Back, manual lymph drainage in, 70-74
Bainbridge reflex, 34
Bandages, use in complete decongestive therapy, 97-99
Blood capillaries
  anatomy of, 28
  fluid exchange within, 16-27
    in arterial and venous branches, 20-21
    concentration equalization in, 16
    concentration gradient in, 16, 17
    diffusion mechanisms of, 16-17
    fluid reabsorption, 21, 22
    hindered diffusion in, 16-17
    osmosis and osmotic pressure mechanisms of, 17-25
    lymphatic serum absorption, 35, 36
    protein circulation in, 25-26
    as semipermeable ultrafilter membrane, 20-21
Blood circulation, purpose of, 16
Blood circulation system, comparison with lymph vessel
  system, 1-2
Blood poisoning (sepsis), 49
Bottlenecks, lymphatic, 86, 96
Breast, manual lymph drainage of, 67
Breast cancer treatment, as lymphedema cause, 11-13
Breathing-coordinated strokes, 82
Buttocks, manual lymph drainage of, 90, 91, 92

C

Cachexia, interstitial pressure in, 23
Calf
  compression-related pump function improvement in,
    98-99
  scoop strokes on, 94, 95
Cancer, lymph node involvement in, 10
Capillaries. *See* Blood capillaries; Lymph capillaries
Capillary blood pressure, 20
  in arterial branches of the blood capillaries, 21
  relationship with net ultrafiltrate, 22, 23
Capillary filtration coefficient, in acute inflammation, 24
Capillary walls, permeability of, 16
Cardiac insufficiency, decompensated, 49
Cardiac output, 34
CBP. *See* Capillary blood pressure
Central strokes, 81
Cervical lymph nodes, 51-64
  accessory nodal chain, 51
  anatomy of, 51-52
  cervicales inferiores
    location of, 52
    manual lymph drainage of, 55, 56
    tributary (drainage) regions of, 14
  cervicales profundi, 51
  cervicales superiores
    location of, 52
    manual lymph drainage of, 55, 56
    tributary (drainage) regions of, 14
  deep, 51, 52
  manual lymph drainage of, 53-64
  superficial, 51, 52
Cervical node chain, manual lymph drainage of, 55-56,
  58, 59
Cheeks, stationary circle strokes on, 61, 63
Chest, manual lymph drainage in, 66-70
Chylus, 6
Cistern, 6
Cisterna chyli, 5, 6
Collector lymph nodes, 10
Collectors
  anatomy and function of, 3, 4-6
  deep (intrafascial), 4-5
  in the extremities, 6
  intestinal, 5
  lymph transport function of, 4
  surface (subcutaneous), 4
Colloidal osmosis, 18